Information Technology Applied to Anesthesiology

Guest Editors

SACHIN KHETERPAL, MD
KEVIN K. TREMPER, MD, PhD

ANESTHESIOLOGY CLINICS

www.anesthesiology.theclinics.com

Consulting Editor
LEE A. FLEISHER, MD, FACC

September 2011 • Volume 29 • Number 3

SAUNDERS an imprint of ELSEVIER, Inc.

W.B. SAUNDERS COMPANY
A Division of Elsevier Inc.

1600 John F. Kennedy Boulevard, Suite 1800 • Philadelphia, PA 19103-2899

http://www.theclinics.com

ANESTHESIOLOGY CLINICS Volume 29, Number 3
September 2011 ISSN 1932-2275, ISBN-13: 978-1-4557-1030-0

Editor: Rachel Glover
Developmental Editor: Donald Mumford

Anesthesiology Clinics (ISSN 1932-2275) is published quarterly by Elsevier Inc., 360 Park Avenue South, New York, NY 10010-1710. Months of issue are March, June, September, and December. Periodicals postage paid at New York, NY and at additional mailing offices. Subscription prices are $141.00 per year (US student/resident), $287.00 per year (US individuals), $351.00 per year (Canadian individuals), $459.00 per year (US institutions), $569.00 per year (Canadian institutions), $198.00 per year (Canadian and foreign student/resident), $398.00 per year (foreign individuals), and $569.00 per year (foreign institutions). To receive student and resident rate, orders must be accompanied by name of affiliated institution, date of term, and the *signature* of program/residency coordinator on institutions letterhead. Orders will be billed at individual rate until proof of status is received. Foreign air speed delivery is included in all *Clinics'* subscription prices. All prices are subject to change without notice. POSTMASTER: Send address changes to *Anesthesiology Clinics,* Elsevier Health Sciences Division, Subscription Customer Service, 3251 Riverport Lane, Maryland Heights, MO 63043. Customer Service (orders, claims, online, change of address): Elsevier Health Sciences Division, Subscription Customer Service, 3251 Riverport Lane, Maryland Heights, MO 63043. Tel:1-800-654-2452 (U.S. and Canada); 314-447-8871 (outside U.S. and Canada). Fax: 314-447-8029. E-mail: journalscustomerservice-usa@elsevier.com (for print support); journalsonlinesupport-usa@elsevier.com (for online support).

Reprints. For copies of 100 or more of articles in this publication, please contact the Commercial Reprints Department, Elsevier Inc., 360 Park Avenue South, New York, NY 10010-1710. Tel.: 212-633-3812; Fax: 212-462-1935; E-mail: reprints@elsevier.com.

Anesthesiology Clinics, is also published in Spanish by McGraw-Hill Inter-americana Editores S. A., P.O. Box 5-237, 06500 Mexico D. F., Mexico.

Anesthesiology Clinics, is covered in *MEDLINE/PubMed (Index Medicus), Current Contents/Clinical Medicine, Excerpta Medica, ISI/BIOMED,* and *Chemical Abstracts.*

Printed and bound by CPI Group (UK) Ltd, Croydon, CR0 4YY

Transferred to Digital Print 2011

Contributors

CONSULTING EDITOR

LEE A. FLEISHER, MD, FACC
Robert D. Dripps Professor and Chair of Anesthesiology and Critical Care, University
of Pennsylvania School of Medicine, Philadelphia, Pennsylvania

GUEST EDITORS

SACHIN KHETERPAL, MD, MBA
Assistant Professor, Principal Investigator, Multicenter Perioperative Outcomes Group,
Department of Anesthesiology, Center for Perioperative Outcomes Research, University
of Michigan Medical School, Ann Arbor, Michigan

KEVIN K. TREMPER, MD, PhD
Robert B. Sweet Professor and Chairman, Department of Anesthesiology, University
of Michigan Medical School, Ann Arbor, Michigan

AUTHORS

ASHLEY ANDERSON, BS
Research Coordinator, Florida Gulf-to-Bay Anesthesiology Associates, Tampa, Florida

ENRICO M. CAMPORESI, MD
Anesthesiologist, Florida Gulf-to-Bay Anesthesiology Associates; Anesthesiologist,
Department of Surgery; Department of Anesthesiology, University of South Florida,
Tampa, Florida

ANDREW DUKATZ, MS
MS-3, University of Maryland School of Medicine, Baltimore, Maryland

RICHARD P. DUTTON, MD, MBA
Executive Director, Anesthesia Quality Institute, Park Ridge, Illinois

JESSE M. EHRENFELD, MD, MPH
Assistant Professor, Massachusetts General Hospital, Boston, Massachusetts; Vanderbilt
University, Nashville, Tennessee

JEFFREY A. GREEN, MD
Vice-Chair, Boyan-Keenan Professor of Anesthesia Safety, Director of Cardiothoracic
Anesthesiology, Department of Anesthesiology, Virginia Commonwealth University
Medical Center, Virginia Commonwealth University, Richmond, Virginia

RACHEL KARLNOSKI, PhD
Research Coordinator, Florida Gulf-to-Bay Anesthesiology Associates; Research
Coordinator, Department of Plastic Surgery, University of South Florida, Tampa, Florida

SACHIN KHETERPAL, MD, MBA
Assistant Professor, Principal Investigator, Multicenter Perioperative Outcomes Group, Department of Anesthesiology, Center for Perioperative Outcomes Research, University of Michigan Medical School, Ann Arbor, Michigan

GRANT H. KRUGER, PhD
Research Investigator, Departments of Anesthesiology and Mechanical Engineering, University of Michigan, Ann Arbor, Michigan

MANDA LAI, MD, MBA
Resident, Center for Perioperative Outcomes Research, Department of Anesthesiology, University of Michigan Medical School, Ann Arbor, Michigan

SIMON LAMBDEN, FRCA
Specialist Registrar Anaesthesia, Academic Clinical Fellow in Anaesthesia, Critical Care and Pain, Department of Anaesthesia Critical Care and Pain, University College London Hospitals, London, United Kingdom

DEVANAND MANGAR, MD
Anesthesiologist and Chief of Staff, Florida Gulf-to-Bay Anesthesiology Associates, Tampa, Florida

BRUCE MARTIN, FRCA
Consultant Anaesthetist, Department of Anaesthesia and Critical Care, The Heart Hospital UCLH NHS Foundation Trust, London, United Kingdom

ANNA MIZZI, MD
Visiting Fellow, CA-1 Anesthesiology Resident, Department of Cardiothoracic and Vascular Anesthesia, San Raffaele Hospital, "Vita-Salute" University, Milan, Italy

BRIAN ROTHMAN, MD
Assistant Professor of Anesthesiology and Medical Director, Perioperative Informatics, Department of Anesthesiology, Vanderbilt University Medical Center, Nashville, Tennessee

WARREN S. SANDBERG, MD, PhD
Professor, Vanderbilt University, Nashville, Tennessee

NIRAV J. SHAH, MD
Assistant Professor, Department of Anesthesiology, Tufts Medical Center, Boston, Massachusetts

SCOTT R. SPRINGMAN, MD
Professor of Anesthesiology (CHS), Anesthesiology Department, University of Wisconsin School of Medicine and Public Health, Madison, Wisconsin

PAUL ST. JACQUES, MD
Associate Professor, Department of Anesthesiology, Vanderbilt University School of Medicine, Nashville, Tennessee

JERRY STONEMETZ, MD
Clinical Associate, Anesthesia and Critical Care Medicine, Johns Hopkins University, Baltimore, Maryland; National Medical Director, Anesthesia Services, Clinical Services Group/Physician Services, Hospital Corporation of America, Nashville, Tennessee

THANH TRAN
Student, Florida Gulf-to-Bay Anesthesiology Associates, Tampa, Florida

KEVIN K. TREMPER, MD, PhD
Robert B. Sweet Professor and Chairman, Department of Anesthesiology, University of Michigan Health System, University of Michigan, Ann Arbor, Michigan

MICHAEL M. VIGODA, MD, MBA
Associate Professor of Anesthesiology, Co-Medical Director, Center for Informatics and Perioperative Management, Clinical Informatics, University of Miami Health System, University of Miami Miller School of Medicine, Miami, Florida

JONATHAN P. WANDERER, MD, MPhil
Resident, Massachusetts General Hospital, Boston, Massachusetts

Contents

Foreword   xiii

Lee A. Fleisher

Preface: Information Technology Comes to Anesthesiology   xv

Sachin Kheterpal and Kevin K. Tremper

SECTION 1: Perioperative Clinical Information Systems

Anatomy of an Anesthesia Information Management System   355

Nirav J. Shah, Kevin K. Tremper, and Sachin Kheterpal

Anesthesia information management systems (AIMS) have become more prevalent as more sophisticated hardware and software have increased usability and reliability. National mandates and incentives have driven adoption as well. AIMS can be developed in one of several software models (Web based, client/server, or incorporated into a medical device). Irrespective of the development model, the best AIMS have a feature set that allows for comprehensive management of workflow for an anesthesiologist. Key features include preoperative, intraoperative, and postoperative documentation; quality assurance; billing; compliance and operational reporting; patient and operating room tracking; and integration with hospital electronic medical records.

Anesthesia Information Management Systems Marketplace and Current Vendors   367

Jerry Stonemetz

This article addresses the brief history of anesthesia information management systems (AIMS) and discusses the vendors that currently market AIMS. The current market penetration based on the information provided by these vendors is presented and the rationale for the purchase of AIMS is discussed. The considerations to be evaluated when making a vendor selection are also discussed.

Clinical Research Using an Information System: The Multicenter Perioperative Outcomes Group   377

Sachin Kheterpal

Clinical research using electronic medical record (EMR) data is an emerging source of scientific progress. Increasingly, researchers are using retrospective observational data acquired from EMRs as the substrate for their clinical research into comorbidities, procedures, situations, and outcomes that have historically presented significant challenges. Although EMR data collection is perceived to require fewer resources than manual chart review, there are many specific regulatory, privacy, data quality, and technique issues unique to clinical research using EMR data. This article discusses the use of EMRs for observational research.

Real-Time Alerts and Reminders Using Information Systems   389

Jonathan P. Wanderer, Warren S. Sandberg, and Jesse M. Ehrenfeld

> Adoption of information systems throughout the hospital environment has enabled the development of real-time physiologic alerts and clinician reminder systems. These clinical tools can be made available through the deployment of anesthesia information management systems (AIMS). Creating usable alert systems requires understanding of technical considerations. Various successful implementations are reviewed, encompassing cost reduction, improved revenue capture, timely antibiotic administration, and postoperative nausea and vomiting prophylaxis. Challenges to the widespread use of real-time alerts and reminders include AIMS adoption rates and the difficulty in choosing appropriate areas and approaches for information systems support.

Shortcomings and Challenges of Information System Adoption   397

Michael M. Vigoda, Brian Rothman, and Jeffrey A. Green

> The number of institutions implementing AIMS is increasing. Shortcomings in the design and implementation of EMRs have been associated with unanticipated consequences, including changes in workflow. These have often resulted from the carryover of paper-based documentation practices into an electronic environment. The new generation of mobile devices allows providers to have situational awareness of multiple care sites simultaneously, possibly allowing for improved proactive decision making. Although potentially facilitating safer anesthetic supervision, technologic and cultural barriers remain. Security, quality of information delivery, regulatory issues, and return on investment will continue as challenges in implementing and maintaining this new technology.

Creating a Real Return-on-Investment for Information System Implementation: Life After HITECH   413

Manda Lai and Sachin Kheterpal

> In 2010, the Centers for Medicare and Medicaid Services (CMS) published its final rule describing plans for incentivizing eligible professionals (EPs) and eligible hospitals to become meaningful users of electronic health record (EHR) technology using funds provided by the Health Information Technology for Economic and Clinical Health (HITECH) Act. Beginning in 2011, non-hospital-based EPs can earn monetary benefits for meeting meaningful use criteria through implementation of certified EHR technology. Most anesthesiologists qualify as non-hospital-based EPs under CMS' new hospital-based definition. The authors distill CMS' final rule into its most basic facts and requirements and explain the implications for US anesthesiologists.

Quality Improvement Using Automated Data Sources: The Anesthesia Quality Institute   439

Richard P. Dutton and Andrew DuKatz

> The Anesthesia Quality Institute has created the National Anesthesia Clinical Outcomes Registry to automatically capture electronic data specific to

anesthesia cases. Data come from billing systems, quality management systems, hospital electronic health care records, and anesthesia information management systems. Aggregation of this data will allow for calculation of national and cohort-specific benchmarks for anesthesia outcomes of interest. Provision of this data to anesthesia practitioners through periodic private reports will motivate improvements in the quality of care.

Integration of the Enterprise Electronic Health Record and Anesthesia Information Management Systems

455

Scott R. Springman

Fewer than 5% of anesthesia departments use an electronic medical record (EMR) that is anesthesia specific. Many anesthesia information management systems (AIMS) have been developed with a focus only on the unique needs of anesthesia providers, without being fully integrated into other electronic health record components of the entire enterprise medical system. To understand why anesthesia providers should embrace health information technology (HIT) on a health system–wide basis, this article reviews recent HIT history and reviews HIT concepts. The author explores current developments in efforts to expand enterprise HIT, and the pros and cons of full enterprise integration with an AIMS.

SECTION 2: Computers in Anesthesia

Advanced Integrated Real-Time Clinical Displays

487

Grant H. Kruger and Kevin K. Tremper

Intelligent medical displays have the potential to improve patient outcomes by integrating multiple physiologic signals, exhibiting high sensitivity and specificity, and reducing information overload for physicians. Research findings have suggested that information overload and distractions caused by patient care activities and alarms generated by multiple monitors in acute care situations, such as the operating room and the intensive care unit, may produce situations that negatively impact the outcomes of patients under anesthesia. This can be attributed to shortcomings of human-in-the-loop monitoring and the poor specificity of existing physiologic alarms. Modern artificial intelligence techniques (ie, intelligent software agents) are demonstrating the potential to meet the challenges of next-generation patient monitoring and alerting.

Enhancing Point of Care Vigilance Using Computers

505

Paul St. Jacques and Brian Rothman

Information technology has the potential to provide a tremendous step forward in perioperative patient safety. Through automated delivery of information through fixed and portable computer resources, clinicians may achieve improved situational awareness of the overall operation of the operating room suite and the state of individual patients in various stages of surgical care. Coupling the raw, but integrated, information with decision support and alerting algorithms enables clinicians to achieve high reliability in documentation compliance and response to care protocols. Future studies and outcomes analysis are needed to quantify the degree of benefit of these new components of perioperative information systems.

The Use of Computers for Perioperative Simulation in Anesthesia, Critical Care, and Pain Medicine   521

Simon Lambden and Bruce Martin

Simulation in perioperative anesthesia training is a field of considerable interest, with an urgent need for tools that reliably train and facilitate objective assessment of performance. This article reviews the available simulation technologies, their evolution, and the current evidence base for their use. The future directions for research in the field and potential applications of simulation technology in anesthesia, critical care, and pain medicine are discussed.

SECTION 3: Bonus Articles

Amiodarone Supplants Lidocaine in ACLS and CPR Protocols   535

Anna Mizzi, Thanh Tran, Devanand Mangar, and Enrico M. Camporesi
Edited by Alan D. Kaye

Amiodarone is an antiarrhythmic medication used to treat and prevent certain types of serious, life-threatening ventricular arrhythmias. Amiodarone gained slow acceptance outside the specialized field of cardiac antiarrhythmic surgery because the side-effects are significant. Recent adoption of amiodarone in the ACLS (Advanced Cardiac Life Support) protocol has somewhat popularized this class of antiarrhythmics. Its use is slowly expanding in the acute medicine setting of anesthetics. This article summarizes the use of Amiodarone by anesthesiologists in the operating room and during cardiopulmonary resuscitation.

Voluven, A New Colloid Solution   547

Anna Mizzi, Thanh Tran, Rachel Karlnoski, Ashley Anderson,
Devanand Mangar, and Enrico M. Camporesi
Edited by Alan D. Kaye

Hydroxyethyl starch (HES) 130/0.4 (Voluven, Fresenius/Hospira, Germany) is indicated for the treatment and prophylaxis of hypovolemia. As the Voluven molecule is smaller than those of other available hydroxyethyl starch products, it is associated with less plasma accumulation and can be safely used in patients with renal impairment. Previous studies have demonstrated that Voluven has comparable effects on volume expansion and hemodynamics as other available HES products. Voluven is also associated with fewer effects on coagulation and may be an acceptable alternative to albumin for volume expansion in situations in which other starches are contraindicated secondary to risk of coagulopathy.

Index   557

FORTHCOMING ISSUES

December 2011

Sedation and Analgesia in the ICU:
Pharmacology, Protocolization, and Clinical
Consequences
Pratik Pandharipande, MD, and
E. Wesley Ely, MD, *Guest Editors*

March 2012

Vascular/Transplant Anesthesia
Rae M. Allain, MD, *Guest Editor*

RECENT ISSUES

June 2011

Regional Analgesia and Acute Pain
Management
Sugantha Ganapathy, MBBS, and
Vincent Chan, MD, *Guest Editors*

March 2011

Quality of Anesthesia Care
Mark D. Neuman, MD, and
Elizabeth A. Martinez, MD, *Guest Editors*

December 2010

Perioperative Pharmacotherapy
Alan D. Kaye, MD, PhD, *Guest Editor*

VISIT US ONLINE!
Access your subscription at:
www.theclinics.com

Foreword

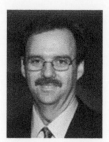

Lee A. Fleisher, MD
Consulting Editor

Technology has always been an important component and interest in the role of the anesthesiologist. It has allowed anesthesiologists to innovate and make undergoing surgery safer through the use of monitoring. While anesthesiologists have been the leaders in the development of electronic medical records, we could become the laggards in the implementation given the incentives created by the HITECH act. Therefore, it is important to understand the issues relevant to the anesthesiologist in the current health care climate. In this issue of *Anesthesiology Clinics*, an excellent group of leaders in the field have written on issues of information systems and computers in anesthesia to inform the reader.

As guest editors for this issue, we are fortunate to have Kevin Tremper, MD, PhD, and Sachin Kheterpal, MD, MBA, both of the University of Michigan. Kevin is currently the Robert B. Sweet Professor and Chair of Anesthesiology. His research initially focused on continuous monitoring of respiratory gases, while more recently he has focused on information systems to manage clinical data for acute perioperative care. He initiated the Multicentered Perioperative Outcomes Group to link academic centers to develop a nationwide database for operative outcomes research. Sachin is currently an Assistant Professor of Anesthesiology. He has been involved in information technology for 20 years and initially worked in the information technology industry before undertaking an internship and residency in anesthesiology. He helped develop the General Electric Medical Systems perioperative information system before joining the Department. Their unique background and experience make them the ideal team to assemble an issue of *Anesthesiology Clinics* on this important topic.

Lee A. Fleisher, MD
University of Pennsylvania School of Medicine
3400 Spruce Street, Dulles 680
Philadelphia, PA 19104, USA

E-mail address:
lee.fleisher@uphs.upenn.edu

Anesthesiology Clin 29 (2011) xiii
doi:10.1016/j.anclin.2011.06.001
1932-2275/11/$ – see front matter

Preface

Information Technology Comes to Anesthesiology

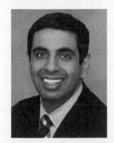 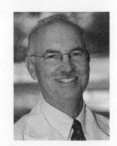

Sachin Kheterpal, MD, MBA   Kevin K. Tremper, MD, PhD
Guest Editors

From the first anesthetic record developed by E. Amory Codman and Harvey Cushing, the field of Anesthesiology has been data driven. Over the first century the vast majority of anesthetic care was documented on a sheet of paper with increasingly dense organized physiologic and treatment data. For that reason the current-day paper anesthesia record usually needs interpretation by an anesthesiologist to be understood by other caregivers. Because the majority of the data we document are high-resolution electronic monitoring data and structured medication and procedure data, our field readily lends itself to computerized documentation. Given this background, it is surprising that it has taken nearly 30 years from the original attempts at developing an electronic anesthesia information system to the point where it is now used in over 50% of academic training programs. In the not too distant future, anesthesia information management systems (AIMS) will be the standard of care.

This issue of *Anesthesiology Clinics* has been divided into two parts: Section I: Perioperative Clinical Information Systems; Section II: Computers in Anesthesia. The first section covers a variety of issues related to the development, design, installation, and applications of AIMS. It is effectively a state of the art on the topic. The second section discusses the application of computers beyond the anesthesia record to the development of integrated alarms and alerts to enhance anesthesia vigilance, quality of care, and the use of computers in echocardiogram simulation for education. The goal of this issue of *Anesthesiology Clinics* is to provide a reference work regarding the application

Anesthesiology Clin 29 (2011) xv–xvi
doi:10.1016/j.anclin.2011.05.011
1932-2275/11/$ – see front matter © 2011 Elsevier Inc. All rights reserved.

of computers for clinical care, teaching, and research. It also provides insight into how these systems fit within the modern hospitals' information technology plan.

Sachin Kheterpal, MD, MBA
Department of Anesthesiology
Center for Perioperative Outcomes Research
University of Michigan Medical School
UH 1H247, Box 0048, 1500 East Medical Center Drive
Ann Arbor, MI 48109, USA

Kevin K. Tremper, MD, PhD
Department of Anesthesiology
University of Michigan Medical School
1500 East Medical Center Drive
Ann Arbor, MI 48109-5048, USA

E-mail addresses:
sachinkh@med.umich.edu (S. Kheterpal)
ktremper@med.umich.edu (K.K. Tremper)

SECTION 1:
Perioperative Clinical Information Systems

Anatomy of an Anesthesia Information Management System

Nirav J. Shah, MD[a],*, Kevin K. Tremper, MD, PhD[b],
Sachin Kheterpal, MD, MBA[c]

KEYWORDS

• AIMS • Anesthesia information system
• Anesthesia record keeper • Clinical information systems

OVERVIEW

Anesthesia information management systems (AIMS) are quickly becoming indispensable components of anesthesiology department operations. Anesthetists, nurses, billing personnel, compliance teams, researchers, and support staff all depend on AIMS capabilities to complete their daily work. Although there is clear evidence that AIMS improve clinical and, occasionally, financial outcomes, some clinicians argue that currently designed systems detract from patient care. For that reason, along with the large expense of software purchase and implementation, the adoption of AIMS has been slower than once expected. Many departments that are using AIMS not only document the patient's clinical course but also comb the immense amounts of data that are generated to answer questions that help improve the quality of care delivered. These departments also work with the commercial vendors and provide invaluable feedback to help improve subsequent generations of the product. AIMS can be a stand-alone product or part of an operating room (OR) management system or a hospital's electronic medical record (EMR). This article gives an overview of the components of AIMS and how they are used. Further details on the implementation and many of the specific functions of AIMS are covered in other articles by Wanderer and colleagues; Kruger and Tremper; Lai and Kheterpal; Vigoda and colleagues elsewhere in this issue.

[a] Department of Anesthesiology, Tufts Medical Center, 800 Washington Street, Box 298, Boston, MA 02111, USA
[b] Department of Anesthesiology, University of Michigan Medical School, 1500 East Medical Center Drive, Ann Arbor, MI 48109-5048, USA
[c] Department of Anesthesiology, Center for Perioperative Outcomes Research, University of Michigan Medical School, UH 1H247, Box 0048, 1500 East Medical Center Drive, Ann Arbor, MI 48109, USA
* Corresponding author.
E-mail address: nshah2@tuftsmedicalcenter.org

Anesthesiology Clin 29 (2011) 355–365
doi:10.1016/j.anclin.2011.05.013
1932-2275/11/$ – see front matter © 2011 Elsevier Inc. All rights reserved.
anesthesiology.theclinics.com

HISTORY OF AIMS

McKesson[1] first described the use of an automatic recording system in 1934. His mechanical contraption recorded tidal volumes, fraction of inspired oxygen (Fio_2), and blood pressure and represented one of the first attempts to avoid the manual transcription of physiologic parameters. Later, Piepenbrink and colleagues[2] described the recording of an anesthetic course using video cameras to document all the information available to the anesthetist while taking care of the patient. Although these attempts helped prove the feasibility of using tools other than paper to create the anesthetic record, none caught on. Modern AIMS started first as intraoperative record keepers. These systems captured physiologic data from the clinical monitors and entered the data in the anesthesia record. This process was supplemented by manually entered information to create the intraoperative record. From these limited beginnings, the breadth of functionality has expanded so that systems now capture the entire perioperative experience, including preoperative, intraoperative, and postoperative care. These systems have also been used on the labor and delivery floor to capture labor and delivery anesthesia, as well as throughout the hospital for acute pain documentation. As these systems have moved from functioning as intraoperative record keepers to workflow managers, departments have started to appreciate benefits in billing, compliance, quality assurance documentation, as well as the expected benefits in legibility, availability, and clinical research.

Several drivers were responsible for the progress in AIMS. First, more sophisticated hardware and software allowed electronic capture of more parameters from medical devices, which in turn allowed for less manual transcription of information and greater user acceptance of AIMS. Second, as anesthesiology departments started to understand gaps in the systems, they worked with AIMS vendors to develop features that allowed for comprehensive workflow management. For example, preoperative clinic, quality assurance, and postoperative care modules were integrated with the intraoperative record keepers. Hospitals began looking to the ORs as revenue generators. ORs can generate a significant part of the health care enterprise's overall earnings, and small changes in perioperative anesthesia processes can lead to large changes in revenue collection. As a result, AIMS began to incorporate more billing functionality. Implementations of AIMS range from those narrow in scope to others in which they function as comprehensive workflow managers, suggesting that although AIMS have been around for many years, much improvement in software, ease of implementation, and affordability needs to be realized.

SOFTWARE COMPONENT OF AIMS

The software used in AIMS can be grouped into 3 architectural categories: medical devices, client/server, and Web based.[3] AIMS that are fundamentally integrated with the anesthesia machine or physiologic monitor are considered medical devices. In these systems, the software user interface is accessed through the device and the software is housed within the device. Advantages of this design include reduced probability of error with recording of hemodynamic parameters and familiar user interface to users with perhaps quicker adoption. The major drawback is that medical devices are significantly more regulated than medical software, which can dramatically slow down development and incorporation of new features.

The second architectural group is the client/server. In this commonly found model, software files are installed on the point-of-care (OR, postanesthesia care unit [PACU], and others) workstation. These files provide instructions on how the software should interact with the user. The files on the workstation (known as the client) also interact with a central computer housing patient data (known as the server) by exchanging patient data. Client server software maintenance can be very resource intensive for hospital information technology (IT) staff because of the need to update all individual workstations every time there is an update in the software. In addition, files loaded on the workstation are susceptible to interactions with files from other programs with unintended consequences. However, advanced system management and automation tools allow for quick distribution and installation of upgrades to workstations to mitigate some of these downsides.[4]

Web-based software uses Web browsers to display the user interface and stores the application instructions in a central computer known as the Web server. Software upgrades are limited to only the Web servers. The workstations are spared because they are only used to house the Web browser. This model is extremely advantageous for large workstation deployments in multiple locations or when the software needs to be accessed remotely (ie, from home). However, currently, user interfaces and features are less mature for Web-based software than client/server, so the interaction between the clinician and software is less robust. In addition, the software may be optimized for a particular Web browser (ie, Microsoft Internet Explorer) and incompatible with others (ie, Mozilla Firefox). The reality is that currently the lines are blurring between the client/server and Web-based models. In addition, combinations of all 3 categories of point-of-care software are possible and may be used to optimize the user's experience and resource requirements of hospital IT staffs.[3]

HARDWARE COMPONENT OF AIMS

Computing hardware at the point of care includes the workstation that the application is accessed from and the mounting equipment used to house the hardware. Several considerations go into choosing the appropriate hardware for each clinical setting in which the software is being used.

1. The hardware should be ergonomic. Mounting equipment should have adequate range of motion to allow the user to interact with the software and simultaneously take care of the patient. Keyboards should be adjustable.
2. The hardware should be compliant with hospital infection control guidelines. Typically, the hospital's infection control team should review all the equipment.
3. The hardware should be durable, resistant to water and other spills, and usable in a variety of temperature settings. The hardware should also be able to withstand the usual bumps and bruises of the OR.
4. The hardware should be procured in an economical manner. Workstation prices are continually dropping, and the hardware purchase is one of the last purchases in an implementation to take advantage of the downward price trajectory of computers.
5. The hardware should be usable in multiple environments, or the hospital should be able to buy equipment specific to each area in which the software will be used.

A few vendors require vendor-specific hardware, either workstations or special keyboards, bar code scanners, or syringe pumps. Hospitals should evaluate the utility of each component of the specialized hardware against cost, support, and training issues.

KEY FEATURES/FUNCTIONALITY OF AIMS

Each commercial vendor has its own specific set of features and functionality. However, there is a significant amount of overlap among the vendors. The most successful implementations allow the clinician to document the patient's clinical course while allowing billing, compliance, and research teams to extract the data for their own purposes. Key features/functionality of AIMS include

- Physiologic device interfaces
- Preoperative history taking and physical examination
- Intraoperative record keeping
- Postoperative documentation
- Billing
- Quality assurance
- Decision support
- Reporting
- Patient tracking
- Configurability
- Integration with institutional EMR.

PHYSIOLOGIC DEVICE INTERFACES

Among the most critical features of AIMS is its ability to automatically interface data from the medical devices into the intraoperative record. Interfaces are software and hardware that allow one system to communicate with another. Without device interfaces, the user would be required to manually type in all the physiologic data into the system to create the anesthetic record. Moreover, intraoperative records generated by AIMS with device interfaces have been shown to be more accurate than handwritten records and, therefore, more useful for review and quality assurance purposes.[5]

Devices commonly interfaced to AIMS include physiologic monitors, anesthesia machines, ventilators, bispectral index monitors, and continuous cardiac output monitors. Less commonly interfaced devices include heart/lung bypass machines and infusion pumps. Basic hemodynamic variables such as blood pressure, heart rate, and pulse oximetry must absolutely be interfaced. Other useful parameters include gas analyzer data such as inspired and expired inhalational anesthetic concentrations, Fio_2, and end-tidal carbon dioxide. Ventilator data, such as tidal volume, respiratory rate, and peak pressures, should also be sent to the AIMS.

Physiologic device interface implementations typically leverage existing monitoring networks that were created to provide a central viewing area for waveforms (such as electrocardiogram) and vital signs from multiple locations. Each of the medical devices in the anesthesia cockpit is connected to specialized hardware, such as Unity ID (General Electric Health care) or Capsule Terminal Server (Capsule), or to a workstation containing specialized software. This hardware or workstation connects the devices and transmits information to the monitoring server. The physiologic device interface server copies information from the monitoring server and places it into the AIMS database. If the monitors also display information from other devices (such as anesthesia machines) and that information is transmitted over the monitoring network, then the interface server can copy information from these other devices as well. If there are devices that are not connected to the monitoring network, then the data from those devices must be copied into a local processing device (usually a personal computer). This device sends the patient information to a central database server, which then copies it into the AIMS. If there is no monitoring network at all, then all devices must interface into the AIMS at the point of care. Then, all patient information is sent from the client to the server.

PREOPERATIVE RECORD

Well-designed preoperative modules of AIMS are able to manage the multiple scenarios in which preoperative information is collected, such as surgeon's offices, via phone triage or a preoperative clinic, or on the morning of surgery. In the best implementations, much of the information for the history taking and physical examination is collected from other sources, including previous anesthesia history and physical examinations, and presented to the anesthetist for review. The anesthetist can then spend less time collecting information and more time analyzing it and producing an anesthetic plan.

Preoperative documentation can be divided into several categories:

1. Patient demographics: examples include name, gender, and date of birth. This information is usually interfaced from hospital registration systems or OR scheduling systems.
2. Preoperative testing: includes laboratory tests, electrocardiography, radiography, and echocardiography. Interfacing of preoperative testing data is highly variable among implementations and depends on several factors, including the technical ability of the testing systems to interface with AIMS and vice versa. Just as important is the model of patient care. If the preoperative testing is done at a facility completely unrelated to the OR facility, then it may not be feasible to electronically exchange information.
3. Allergies and medications: if the information is automatically captured from other sources, then the anesthetist must verify these before completing the history taking and physical examination. If not, then the system should be designed to easily input allergies and medications.
4. Past medical history and review of systems including previous surgeries and problems with anesthesia: usually follows a systems approach. If manually entered, then systems typically provide multiple methods to input the information, such as selecting from a list of choices, typing information into a text box, or choosing a default option (for example, within normal limits). If the AIMS have the ability to automatically capture information that was previously entered, then the information must be verified before becoming part of the preoperative history.
5. Physical examination: vital signs, height, and weight. This information can be interfaced from the physiologic monitor and/or captured from the initial nursing assessment. In addition, AIMS can provide useful tools to automatically take information from the history and physical examination and calculate derived values such as body mass index or antiemetic scores.
6. Procedure information including surgeon and proposed operation; this information should be automatically captured from the OR scheduling system. If not, AIMS typically allow users to select from a list of choices.
7. Anesthetic assessment and plan: including the American Society of Anesthesiologists class, airway management, monitoring, and patient discussion acknowledgment.

INTRAOPERATIVE RECORD

The intraoperative component of the AIMS must allow for quick and accurate documentation (**Box 1**). Screen layout must be well thought out, methodology of data input should be intuitive, and the overall ergonomics should be conducive to the multitasking that occurs in the OR environment.[6] Although much of the clinical information is automatically captured from the physiologic monitors or other medical devices into the intraoperative record, there are also usually parameters that need to be manually

---

Box 1
Categories of user-entered documentation with selected examples

Required documentation for billing or regulatory guidelines

- Anesthesia and surgical times
- Machine check
- Confirmation of case, history and physical review, and NPO
- Time-out confirming patient, case, and side with surgical and nursing colleagues
- Timing of antibiotic dosing
- Patient disposition such as transport to PACU or surgical intensive care unit

Routine and nonroutine clinical events that occur during the surgical case

- Induction events such as laryngoscopic view
- Patient positioning
- Intravenous lines placed
- Adverse events such as bronchospasm and laryngospasm

Notes or forms completed by the anesthetist during the case

- Documentation for procedures such as arterial lines or central venous lines
- Difficult airway letters for patients
- Acute pain service consults for patient-controlled analgesia management or patients with chronic pain

Clinical or physiologic data that may not be captured by the physiologic monitors

- Train of 4 counts
- Fresh gas flows
- Eyes checked

Medications/fluids/infusions/blood products

- Bolus medications
- Fluids, with amounts given and rates
- Drug infusions such as vasopressors or narcotics
- Blood products

Case times

- Anesthesia start/end
- Surgery start/end

---

entered because of either hardware or software limitations. Specific items are required for quality assurance or billing reasons and must be documented by the user in the anesthetic record. AIMS can be used to increase the rate of documentation completion of these items.[7] However, there are also instances in which, despite the implementation of AIMS, incomplete documentation persisted in the anesthesia record.[8]

POSTOPERATIVE DOCUMENTATION

Postoperative documentation consists of the hand off from anesthetist to PACU nurse, whereby a report is given and the initial set of postoperative vital signs is documented. It also consists of the postoperative anesthesia note. AIMS need to have postoperative functionality to allow the user to document the entire anesthetic course in a single system.

STAFF AND BILLING INFORMATION

AIMS can be extremely useful to billing and compliance teams by ensuring all items required for billing are properly recorded and that all compliance measures are accounted for. Many institutions that use AIMS have been able to significantly improve billing. Spring and colleagues[9] were able to reduce their percentage of unbillable records from 1.31% to 0.04% and increase annual revenue by $400,000.

Staff Concurrency Checks

Many anesthesia care models have several anesthetic caregivers involved in a particular case. Anesthesiologists may be supervising multiple nurses or residents, breaks are given, and responsibility of care is transferred from one anesthetist to another. Anesthetists are expected to accurately and reliably sign in and out of cases as they are associated or disassociated with them. However, on a typically busy day in an OR, time-related documentation mistakes commonly occur, which can have multiple adverse ramifications. Specific institutions, as well as insurance companies, have rules on the number of cases that can be simultaneously supervised by an anesthesiologist. AIMS can keep track of the cases that each anesthetist is associated with and perform real-time concurrency checks so that no caregiver is associated with more cases than is allowed at any given time. This function saves the billing team a time-consuming task and reduces the possibility of rejected bills; furthermore, it allows anesthesia departments to be compliant with institutional policies.

Automatic Charge Capture

Anesthesia charge capture is a complex process, involving not only the complexity of the procedure but also the patient's clinical condition and the time spent with the patient. Every single anesthetic is a unique charge, and AIMS can provide significant financial upside by ensuring all charges are captured.[10] AIMS can reduce the time spent by the billing staff in generating a charge by automatically abstracting the necessary billing information from the anesthetic record. This information includes

- Patient identifying information
- Provider information
- Anesthesia times (anesthesia start and end)
- Procedure information (complete procedure and accompanying diagnosis).

QUALITY ASSURANCE

Electronic documentation of the anesthetic record can greatly facilitate documentation of adverse events. Benson and colleagues[11] demonstrated that manual charting underreports the true number of adverse events. An integrated quality assurance module should allow users to document adverse events. In addition, users should be able to automatically send events documented on the anesthetic record to the quality assurance module to prevent duplicate documentation.

DECISION SUPPORT

Decision support is any aid that reduces the possibility of error or increases the probability of making the correct decision. Decision support functionality in AIMS can help standardize clinical practices, reduce errors of omission, and prevent anesthetists from delivering harmful medication or medication doses.[12]

Case Templates

Cardiac anesthesia cases are managed differently from routine hysterectomies. Intra-operative templates take these into account and enable best practices to be followed. Templates can significantly help institutions follow practice guidelines. Placing antibiotic dosing on case templates, in addition to physician-specific reminders, increased compliance with antibiotic administration from 69% to 92% in one study.[13]

Alerts and Reminders

Alerts and reminders are important tools to help ensure the completeness of documentation and adherence to standard of care. When used judiciously, these alerts and reminders guide the user to do the right thing without interfering with the speed of documentation. When used with reckless abandon, they slow down the user and cause extreme angst and rebellion. Alerts can take several forms, including

- Pop-up windows in the AIMS
- Pager or e-mail messages
- Highlighting or bolding of certain items within the AIMS.

These features in AIMS have been used time and time again to address areas in which institutions needed to be more compliant. There have been many examples of improved administration of prophylactic antibiotics with AIMS using alerts and reminders.[13–15] Wax and colleagues[14] studied the administration of antibiotic prophylaxis in patients before and after the implementation of a visual reminder. The investigators found that compliance increased from 82.4% to 89.1% with the reminder. Sandberg and colleagues[16] used automated text messaging to reduce missing allergy documentation from 30% to 8%. Kheterpal and colleagues[17] developed an automated reminder system for peripheral arterial catheter placement in the ORs. The experimental group received pager alerts when the arterial line documentation was not completed in a timely manner. During the 2-month trial, the group that received pager reminders had a significantly higher documentation rate (88% vs 75%, $P<.001$). When all users were sent reminders, the documentation rate increased to 99%, which resulted in a net increase in reimbursement of $40,500.

REPORTING FOR QUALITY IMPROVEMENT, COMPLIANCE, OR RESEARCH PURPOSES

Institutions implement AIMS for many reasons: increased operational efficiency, adoption of best practices, and reduced liability. They also implement AIMS to be able to comply with local and national regulatory requirements. The Centers for Medicare and Medicaid Services (CMS) announced to great publicity that it would provide bonus payments to providers that could report increased quality of care through a variety of measures. Initially, CMS asked for voluntary reporting on several quality measures. For anesthesiologists, these included timely administration of prophylactic antibiotics and prevention of catheter-related bloodstream infections.[18,19] Robust reporting functionality is crucial to meeting these objectives. Analyzing clinical, financial, and operational metrics across patients provide data-driven justification for process changes. The resulting cost savings and improvement in charge capture and patient outcomes can provide justification for the high cost of implementing AIMS.

PATIENT TRACKING

Patient tracking components of AIMS take all the scheduling information and clinical documentation entered to create a real-time view showing the progress of the day's cases. Tracking features are typically reliant on information generated from the OR management information system. The initial starting point is the OR schedule of the day. The progress of each case is shown by a visual cue triggered by a documentation event in the OR. For example, selecting "In Room" in the intraoperative component of the AIMS when a patient is taken to the OR automatically changes the color of the case as seen on the patient tracker. In this way, the progress of cases becomes readily transparent and changes can be made to facilitate patient throughput. Schedule changes, such as room changes or case cancellations, are automatically updated on the patient tracker. Information such as anesthesia personnel and anesthesia times can also be reflected on the patient tracker. Many ORs currently have large dry-erase boards used as patient trackers. The digital patient tracker automates this whiteboard, enhances it by adding information provided from the OR in real time, and distributes the information to any workstation that is able to view the tracker. This distribution of information allows all users to participate in enhancing patient throughput.

INTEGRATION WITH INSTITUTIONAL EMRs

AIMS are just one of many software systems used in an institution. These multitudes of systems were typically implemented over long periods and have varying levels of inter-operability. These systems include the hospital EMR, computerized provider order entry, laboratory information systems, radiology systems, document imaging systems, and many others. The anesthetic record needs to become part of the EMR so that other providers can view it when necessary. Given that AIMS are not typically fully integrated parts of the hospital EMR, there has to be an interface built between them. Most EMRs and document imaging systems are able to accept an exported image of the anesthetic record as long as it is in a supported format (portable document format [PDF], tagged image file format [TIFF], and other formats). AIMS should be able to send a document or image of the anesthetic record to the EMR. The EMR then provides a method for other providers to access and view the record from sites other than the OR where the AIMS are installed.

Equally important as accessing the anesthetic record from the EMR is accessing patient information while the anesthetist is using the AIMS. There are several ways this can be accomplished, and the methodology depends on many factors, such as the interfacing capability of the AIMS and institutional software systems, institutional philosophy regarding access of its systems, and breadth of deployment of other systems within an institution. One method is to interface the AIMS with key clinical information systems needed by users. In this scenario, laboratory, pathology, and departmental testing information; dictated notes such as history and physical and discharge summaries; radiology images; medication administration; and electronic orders would be interfaced to the AIMS for viewing by the anesthetist. A second scenario is using a single logon architecture with patient context to automatically launch other hospital systems such as the hospital EMR with the same patient displayed to avoid having to search for the patient again. This scenario has the advantage of requiring less interfacing work but requires the user to be familiar with the other application that is opened. A third grim scenario is that the user has to manually open each system, including the paper chart, separately to find the necessary clinical information. The reality is that because the transition to EMRs is a long journey, clinicians use combinations of all 3 scenarios to retrieve clinical information in many institutions and to find a way to balance efficiency with retrieving all the necessary information to take care of the patient.

SUMMARY

AIMS are complex expensive systems that take great amounts of effort to buy and implement. However, the advantages of a legible easily accessible record that allows the clinical team and support services to use the system to complete work safely and efficiently have ensured that these systems will become more prevalent in the coming years.

REFERENCES

1. McKesson EI. The technique of recording the effects of gas-oxygen mixtures, pressures, rebreathing and carbon-dioxide, with a summary of the effects. Anesth Analg 1934;13(1):1–14.
2. Piepenbrink JC, Cullen JI Jr, Stafford TJ. A real-time anesthesia record keeping system using video. J Clin Eng 1990;15(5):391–3.
3. Kheterpal S. Architecture. In: Stonemetz J, Ruskin K, editors. Anesthesia informatics. 1st edition. New York (NY): Springer; 2008. p. 147–65.
4. Thick client/thin client. Available at: http://www.wikipedia.com. Accessed June 9, 2010.
5. Thrush DN. Are automated anesthesia records better? J Clin Anesth 1992;4(5): 386–9.
6. Shah N, O'Reilly M. Intraoperative charting requirements. In: Stonemetz J, Ruskin K, editors. Anesthesia informatics. 1st edition. New York (NY): Springer; 2008. p. 191–208.
7. Vigoda MM, Gencorelli F, Lubarsky DA. Changing medical group behaviors: increasing the rate of documentation of quality assurance events using an anesthesia information system. Anesth Analg 2006;103(2):390–5.
8. Driscoll WD, Columbia MA, Peterfreund RA. An observational study of anesthesia record completeness using an anesthesia information management system. Anesth Analg 2007;104(6):1454–61.
9. Spring SF, Sandberg WS, Anupama S, et al. Automated documentation error detection and notification improves anesthesia billing performance. Anesthesiology 2007;106(1):157–63.
10. Reeves C, Stonemetz J. Automated charge capture. In: Stonemetz J, Ruskin K, editors. Anesthesia informatics. 1st edition. New York (NY): Springer; 2008. p. 269–94.
11. Benson M, Junger A, Fuchs C, et al. Using an anesthesia information management system to prove a deficit in voluntary reporting of adverse events in a quality assurance program. J Clin Monit Comput 2000;16(3):211–7.
12. Vigoda MM, O'Reilly M, Gencorelli FJ, et al. Decision support. In: Stonemetz J, Ruskin K, editors. Anesthesia informatics. 1st edition. New York (NY): Springer; 2008. p. 295–310.
13. O'Reilly M, Talsma A, VanRiper S, et al. An anesthesia information system designed to provide physician-specific feedback improves timely administration of prophylactic antibiotics. Anesth Analg 2006;103(4):908–12.
14. Wax DB, Beilin Y, Levin M, et al. The effect of an interactive visual reminder in an anesthesia information management system on timeliness of prophylactic antibiotic administration. Anesth Analg 2007;104(6):1462–6.

15. St Jacques P, Sanders N, Patel N, et al. Improving timely surgical antibiotic prophylaxis redosing administration using computerized record prompts. Surg Infect (Larchmt) 2005;6(2):215–21.
16. Sandberg WS, Sandberg EH, Seim AR, et al. Real-time checking of electronic anesthesia records for documentation errors and automatically text messaging clinicians improves quality of documentation. Anesth Analg 2008;106(1): 192–200.
17. Kheterpal S, Gupta R, Blum JM, et al. Electronic reminders improve procedure documentation compliance and professional fee reimbursement. Anesth Analg 2007;104(3):592–7.
18. Physicians quality reporting initiative. Available at: http://www.cms.gov/PQRI. Accessed June 9, 2010.
19. Sandberg WS. Anesthesia information management systems: almost there. Anesth Analg 2008;107(4):1100–2.

Anesthesia Information Management Systems Marketplace and Current Vendors

Jerry Stonemetz, MD[a,b],*

KEYWORDS

- AIMS vendors • Market penetration • Vendor selection criterion

Anesthesia information management systems (AIMS) is a relatively new moniker for a technology that has been in existence for more than 20 years. The original label for systems that captured clinical data from patient monitors during an anesthetic started as simple record keepers, and hence the original acronym of ARK (anesthesia record keeping) was used to signify systems such as DAME (Duke Anesthesia Monitoring Equipment) created at Duke University and ARKIVE (Anesthesia Record Keeper Integrating Voice Recognition), a product from Diatek. The DAME product at Duke University was possibly the first authentic application for capturing patient data during an anesthetic. This software application was the first successful implementation of a clinical system that involved a direct interface to the clinical monitors to electronically capture data on patient vital signs. This initial product, developed in the research laboratories, was only capable of being implemented in a few of the operating rooms and used by a limited number of clinicians; however, it was a seminal moment in the history of anesthesia electronic records. Concomitantly, on the other side of the continent, efforts from the inimitable Ty Smith at the University of San Diego resulted in the creation of a voice-activated software system that allowed anesthesia providers to input discreet data elements into a database while performing anesthesia. Ultimately, deemed to be an inferior user interface (primarily because of an artifact arising from surgeons insisting on discussing nonrelevant information during the case), his pioneering research led to the private enterprise Diatek picking up this application and pushing it to market. In fact, the first commercial product ARKIVE was derived from the voice-activated application designed by Dr Smith (Dan Pettus, Product Manager at Diatek, personal communication, 2010).

[a] Anesthesia and Critical Care Medicine, Johns Hopkins University, Baltimore, MD 21287, USA
[b] Anesthesia Services, Clinical Services Group/Physician Services, Hospital Corporation of America, Nashville, TN 37027, USA
* Anesthesia and Critical Care Medicine, Johns Hopkins University, Baltimore, MD 21287.
E-mail address: Jstonemetz@jhmi.edu

Anesthesiology Clin 29 (2011) 367–375
doi:10.1016/j.anclin.2011.05.009
1932-2275/11/$ – see front matter © 2011 Elsevier Inc. All rights reserved.

Although named for the voice-activation functionality of ARKIVE, the original product was in fact based on a touch screen user interface. Coming to market with a revolutionary new technology, ARKIVE made an initial impact by getting contracts initially at Vero Beach Hospital, followed by Duke University and Fitchburg Hospital in New Hampshire. These 3 implementations were solely based on the single-minded compulsion of true pioneers in this space. These pioneers were Frank Block of Vero Beach, Ted Stanley of Duke University, and David Edsall of Fitchburg Hospital. The collective wisdom and current industry owes these 3 evangelists a great deal for their insight and fortitude. Although recognized even today for the creative genius of fast keyboard entries and creation of template-generated documentation, ARKIVE succumbed to the market reality of the fallibility of servicing a product when the market is not ready.

As more commercial systems became available, companies began attempting to differentiate themselves by providing a more comprehensive solution than simply generating an anesthesia record, and these products were labeled anesthesia information systems. Eventually, vendors began to seize on the concept of using this clinical data in an effort to allow the anesthesia group the ability to manage their environment, and, hence, they began to market their products as AIMS. Successive companies invested significantly in this new technology, including companies such as LifeLog, which was built on the OS2 operating system from IBM and designed with help from Bill Merritt at Hopkins; CompuRecord, created by a true genius Chester Phillips (both anesthesiologist and programmer); and even my old company, AIMCare, which was the first to introduce a Windows graphical user interface. Ironically, only Dr Phillips' system is still in use today in the current (and much altered) iteration sold as the Phillips system (no relation of inventor to company).

All these vendors envisioned that the market was radically expand and they would soon be generating buckets of cash and profitability. I remember very well promising to multiple investors and boards that "this was the year." That was almost 20 years ago, and AIMS are still only fractionally adopted by the profession. And why is that?

My personal view is that the adoption has been retarded by 3 primary issues:

1. Usability: first and foremost, anesthesia providers live in a production pressure environment and absolutely tolerate nothing that slows them down or impedes their ability to move rapidly from one case to another. It is difficult to improve on pen and paper. For those who have used some of the more sophisticated systems of today, this is no longer a major issue. Most vendor systems of today have the ability to allow templates and documentation from pick lists that actually do enhance the ability to document the anesthetic experience. Anyone who has used AIMS will also attest to the absurdity of charting vital signs every 5 minutes. What a colossal waste of time for highly trained anesthesia providers to spend most of their time manually charting numbers on a piece of paper! The system captures all these parameters, and the providers simply annotate updates and unique scenarios. It is arguable that the user interface has advanced to the point that this rationale is no longer valid.

2. This record will be used against me: clearly the automatic capture of every vital sign gives most anesthetists pause. Some cases involve blood pressures that are deemed to be extremely low, yet these patients all seem to do well despite the horrible numbers. Anesthesia providers are primarily concerned that these actual recordings will be used against them if one of their patients wakes up with an adverse outcome. In reality, what is known is that these systems in fact help protect providers unless they are reading the Wall Street Journal and not paying attention to detail. Feldman[1] provided data on how these systems actually benefit anesthesia

providers' defensives from the claims database. Now, granted, it is also incumbent on anesthesia providers to actually do as they are charting, as has been illustrated by Vigoda and Lubarsky.[2]

3. Return on investment: this is likely the most significant issue that is currently impeding acceptance of this technology. Although the scope of this topic is too extensive for this article, suffice to say that a price tag of $25,000 per anesthesia location is difficult to justify to hospital administrators when the industry has not done a sufficient job of illustrating a real return on investment. I discuss frequently that the new driving force in adoption of these systems will be in reporting quality indicators surrounding the surgical experience[3]; however, it is not just these systems that are required but a comprehensive change in the mindset of the anesthesia provider to accept responsibility and ownership of all quality indicators involving surgical patients. Only then will these systems become an effective tool that allows these providers to demonstrate to the hospital administrators that they are capable of not only delivering a quality anesthetic but also providing documentation and proof of that delivery.

SO WHERE ARE WE TODAY

Multiple studies have illustrated that AIMS provide better documentation, better solutions for quality improvement, and possibly safer patient care, yet market penetration is still very low. I recently published an article in the *ASA Newsletter* (represented with permission of the editorial staff of the *ASA Newsletter*) that outlines my recent investigation of this issue, and I paraphrase much of the article in the following.[4] This past year, I updated these figures in preparation for publication of a white paper on AIMS sanctioned by the American Society of Anesthesia under the auspices of the Committee on Information Management, which is due for publication this year (in press).

The American Recovery and Reinvestment Act of 2009 included provisions to advance health care information technology (IT) under the Health Information Technology for Economic and Clinical Health (see the article by Lai and Kheterpal elsewhere in this issue for further exploration of this topic). There is a universal movement toward electronic health records (EHRs), and many argue that the return on investment of these systems needs to factor in the ability to measure and demonstrate quality care. New evidence is beginning to be produced that, in fact, higher-quality metrics are associated with hospitals that achieve a high level of adoption of integrated EHRs (**Fig. 1**).[5]

AIMS have had an excruciatingly slow rate of adoption since the first systems came on the market during the late 1980s. Published in *Anesthesia and Analgesia* in 2008, it was reported that 44% of academic institutions were either implementing or planning on implementing AIMS, which illustrated an inflection point in the adoption of AIMS by academic centers.[6] However, there are little data on the roughly 5000 US hospitals with surgical suites as reported by the American Hospital Association (AHA; http://www.aha.org/aha/resource-center/Statistics-and-Studies/fast-facts.html American Hospital Association Web site; last accessed on July 19, 2010) that would be potential candidates for AIMS. It is unclear how many community hospitals are even considering AIMS. In preparation for this publication, I contacted 13 AIMS vendors who are actively marketing products and segregated these vendors into 3 categories. The first was vendors whose products were incorporated into clinical monitors or anesthesia machines. The second group was vendors who sold operating room management systems, and the third group was vendors who sold exclusively AIMS. **Table 1** lists currently available vendors, their products, and corporate URLs.

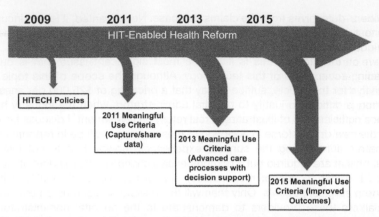

Fig. 1. Health information technology–enabled health reform. Meaningful Use Workgroup, Health IT Policy Committee. HITECH, Health Information Technology for Economic and Clinical Health. (*Courtesy of* Dr Jonathan Perlin, CMO HCA, Chair Health IT Standards Committee, HHS, and the editorial staff of the ASA Newsletter.)

Table 1
Listing of current AIMS vendors and products

Vendor	Product	URL
General Electric	Centricity Anesthesia	http://www.gehealthcare.com/euen/iis/products/anesthesia/iis_anesthesia.html
Drager	Innovian Anesthesia	http://www.draeger.com/US/en_US/products/medical_monitoring/patient_data_management/mon_innovian_anesthesia.jsp?showBackButton=true
Philips	CompuRecord	http://www.healthcare.philips.com/in/products/patient_monitoring/products/icip/anesthesia/index.wpd
Picis	Anesthesia Manager	http://www.picis.com/solutions/perioperative-services/anesthesia-manager.aspx
McKesson	Anesthesia Care	http://www.mckesson.com/en_us/McKesson.com/For%2BHealthcare%2BProviders/Hospitals/Surgical%2BSolutions/McKesson%2BAnesthesia%2BCare.html
Surgical Information Systems	Anesthesia	http://www.sisfirst.com/products/module/SIS-Anesthesia/
Cerner	SurgiNet Anesthesia Management	https://store.cerner.com/items/230
Epic	Anesthesia Information Management System	http://www.epic.com/software-ancillaries.php
Merge	AIMS DS	http://www.merge.com/products/docusys/aims/index.aspx
IMDSoft	Metavision	http://www.imd-soft.com/anesthesia
Acuitec	Gaschart	http://acuitec.com/solutions-for/anesthesia/
Plexus	Anesthesia Touch	http://www.plexusis.com/products.aspx
Cosalient	Healthware	http://www.cosalient.com/

Tables 2–4 report the market penetration of these 3 groups. The vendors were asked to provide the number of live AIMS sites, the number under implementation, and the number under contract. This third group is presumed to represent hospitals that have purchased AIMS but not yet begun to stage the implementation.

Looking at the total number of systems under contract, it could be assumed (providing the reporting data are valid) that a new inflection point has been reached in the market with a market penetration of 27%. However, the real story is most likely only looking at the current live sites and sites under implementation because it is not clear how many of the contract group will really install. This group represents a market penetration of 14.8%, which is still a significant increase from previously reported figures. This increase in penetration is thought to be a result of a de facto movement toward EHRs and not because undisputable evidence of a return on investment has been demonstrated. Recent studies looking at market adoption of computerized physician order entry systems using the Bass model of predicting market penetration have predicted that the tipping point (>80% market penetration) is unlikely to occur before 2025 at current adoption rates.[7] It is unrealistic to presume that AIMS will have a more rapid adoption rate, but it is encouraging that there is finally a market penetration of more than 10%. As found with other EHR implementations, full integration with other clinical systems is likely the barrier that is to be overcome before the truly definable value of AIMS is seen and rapid adoption by providers takes place.

The limitations to these data are that self-reported data are accepted from vendors with no method of validating this information. It is possible that vendors reported larger numbers of sites than are currently fully operational. In addition, it is perceived that the vendors likely reported multiple facilities as separate sites even if they were associated with the same institution. From the anesthesia provider's perspective, these facilities can be considered as individual because the number of hospitals reported by the AHA also lists these types of settings as individual facilities.

NON-AIMS VENDORS

There are also several vendors who have created products that are marketed to anesthesiologists, which, however, are not fully functioning AIMS. Although a thorough description of these vendors is not provided in this article, there are some points that are worth mentioning because these vendors do have products that particular customers may think have value. Typically because these products have less functionality than AIMS, they are usually much less expensive or less complex to implement and maintain. Table 5 lists some of these vendors with a brief description of their products.

VENDOR CHOICES

Most of those who pursue a vendor selection are faced with the absolute certainty that the choice is heavily influenced by the hospital administration because ultimately it is

Table 2				
Vendors who sell AIMS integrated with clinical monitors or anesthesia machines				
Vendor	**Number of Live AIMS Sites (United States)**	**Number Under Implementation**	**Number Under Contract**	**Number Sold/ Not Begun Implementation**
GE/Philips/ Draeger	197	76	273	0

Table 3
Vendors who sell AIMS integrated with operating room management systems

Vendor	Number of Live AIMS Sites (United States)	Number Under Implementation	Number Under Contract	Number Sold/ Not Begun Implementation
GE[a]/Picis/McKesson/ SIS/Cerner/Epic	216	138	1099	741

[a] GE is counted twice (but only once in the aggregate number of sites).

the hospital's dollars that are used to purchase these systems. These administrators typically look to the Chief Information Officer (CIO) for feedback, and, almost universally, these individuals prefer a single-vendor solution. The rationale for their preference should be self-evident and primarily involves the perception that a single source yields better integration and support. In reality, many of these single-vendor solutions are in fact applications coupled together from disparate companies and purchased by the single vendor. Regardless, the argument is still made that, eventually, these products achieve a higher degree of integration.

Alternatively, the user frequently focuses on the best-of-breed vendor for whom they perceive a higher degree of functionality and usability. It has not been uncommon for hospitals to purchase or acquire AIMS only for the anesthesia group to refuse to use the product.

Consequently, these decisions need a thorough discussion of all stakeholders, and, depending on the vendor, it may be prudent to seek a best-of-breed solution. For most users, any system that does not facilitate the start of a new case and easy documentation of the typical charting requirements will not be well received. The ability to accurately capture and enhance professional fee charge capture, for example, may be an extremely high priority for the anesthesia group but has little to no value to the hospital unless there is a significant subsidy being paid. There are, however, clear indications that the most value to be received from AIMS results from a comprehensive integration to existing hospital and patient data. The ability to automatically import patient allergies and medications, laboratory test results, and timing of medications given is invaluable to an AIMS user.

PROCESS FOR MAKING A DECISION

For those users who are attempting to make a decision regarding the purchase of AIMS, it would be useful to review the recommendations that were published by a group from New Hampshire who implemented an electronic medical record system.[8] Their recommendations are pertinent to any clinical information system and are briefly outlined in **Table 6**.

Table 4
Vendors who sell exclusively AIMS

Vendor	Number of Live AIMS Sites (United States)	Number Under Implementation	Number Under Contract	Number Sold/ Not Begun Implementation
DocuSys[a]/iMDSoft/Merge (Eko)/Acuitec	55	10	65	3

[a] Since publication of these data, DocuSys has been acquired by Merge.

Table 5
Non-AIMS vendors

Vendor	Product Definition	URL
Shareable Ink	A smart pen and digitized form that allows data capture of discreet data elements from using a pen to document on the form	http://www.shareableink.com
Anescan	A computerized system to generate professional fees	http://www.anescaninc.com
One Medical Passport	A computerized preoperative questionnaire	http://www.onemedicalpassport.com
My Medical File	Patient health record (preoperative) combined with fax and indexing service for all surgical documents	http://www.mmf.com
Quantum	Data collection system for capturing quality data	http://www.quantumcns.com/
ePREOP	An online patient questionnaire that generates preoperative testing recommendations along with patient information	https://www1.epreop.com/

Table 6
Recommendations for selecting an electronic medical record

What is Important	Relevance to AIMS
Functionality	Device interfaces, comprehensive record, charting requirements, charge capture
Implementation/training	IT resources, vendor resources, anesthesia department resources
Interfaces	ADT, operating room scheduling, or laboratory results; costs, resources required, updates
Performance	Network speed, screen changes, number of screens required to document
HIPAA concerns	Access to data, transmission of data, segregation of PHI for anesthesia use
Service level agreement	Clearly defines what vendor is responsible for providing versus hospital resources
Problem resolution	How to escalate an issue for resolution beyond help desk or departmental resource
Data ownership	Who owns the data? The hospital, anesthesia group, or vendor?
Disaster management and recovery	Think Hurricane Katrina. These are mission-critical applications
Disengagement process	In the event of a vendor failure, how to disengage and remain in possession of data and systems

Abbreviations: ADT, admission discharge transfer; HIPAA, Health Insurance Portability and Accountability Act; PHI, public health information.

The investigators also lay out a plan for getting to a decision. The following milestones should be formalized:

- Create a selection team.
- Establish selection criteria (build consensus on priorities); it is important to rank criteria in the event more than one vendor is considered appropriate.
- Develop pro forma strategies, clinical as well as implementation.
- Conduct product demonstrations.
- Distribute request for proposals (RFPs).
- Conduct site visits.
- Make a vendor recommendation.

As described by Muravchick,[9] the selection team should include an anesthesia clinical leader who is the evangelist, an IT implementation project manager, a hospital operating room supervisor (or surrogate) to analyze workflow issues, and an administrator from the executive suite (frequently the CIO). Epstein[10] has provided good descriptions and examples of request for information and RFP.

The final determination of a vendor needs to factor in some specific criteria that may be unique to the environment. These criteria include

1. Current technology: is the system designed on a technology platform that would work in your environment? Many hospital information departments are comfortable with only a limited number of operating systems. Make sure the technology will not be challenging to your IT staff who will likely be necessary for support.
2. Full functionality: does the system have the ability to generate a comprehensive record, in addition to other specifics that may be variable? For example, does the system have the ability to generate professional fees (charge capture), or will the billing office be required to generate fees from a printed anesthesia record? Does the system have the capability to enforce and enhance compliance with proper billing requirements?
3. Applicable for all locations: will this system be able to be implemented and used in remote locations? Obstetric suites? Outpatient facilities?
4. Vendor stability: is the vendor financially stable with good managerial staff? Many of these companies are start-up vendors, and history has demonstrated that most of these vendors do not remain in the market. Make certain you are working with a vendor that has staying power.
5. Compatible environments: does the vendor have customers who are identical to your environment (academic, private community, research, and so forth)?

Once the field of vendors has been narrowed to just a few, then the process should involve an RFP. After review, ideally the list of vendors becomes even smaller, possibly 2 or 3. At this point, it becomes necessary to establish product demonstrations, preferably on-site demonstrations with scripts; PowerPoint presentations should be avoided. The customer needs to drive the system. Eventually, the final stage includes site visits to existing customers. It is essential to see the system in place, making sure that it is being used in all the operating rooms by all providers. Make sure to talk to providers besides the ones introduced by the vendor if possible. The ultimate decision needs to include a financial analysis. Make sure that the net present value is used as well as the manpower needed to assess the true costs of ownership of these systems.

When attempting to make a decision about which vendor to choose, it is important to rank the selection criteria, and the hospital management needs to be included in this ranking process. It may not be possible to arrive at a universal consensus on systems, so it is critical to establish the decision maker in advance in the event of the inability to achieve a consensus. In fact, the selection may actually be decided by which vendor is less of a risk. Ultimately, the success of any of these systems depends in large part on the contracts that are signed between parties. It is advisable to begin negotiating the contract during the sales process; otherwise, the vendor may be less inclined to acquiesce on specific issues.

All these systems involve a change in workflow and behavior. It is vital to have effective change management during the implementation and roll out of these systems. The customer should continue to generate gap analyses during implementation and afterward at regular intervals to make sure that the system continues to provide all the functionality and value that was promised.

SUMMARY

Although AIMS have been in existence for more than 30 years, current market penetration remains low primarily because of resistance based on a poor demonstration of a return on investment. This trend seems to be changing, primarily because of the necessity of reporting on quality metrics and demonstration of compliance with various requirements to demonstrate quality. Anyone anticipating adoption of AIMS should become familiar with the various vendors that are available and become part of the selection process.

REFERENCES

1. Feldman JM. Do anesthesia information systems increase medical malpractice exposure? Results of a survey. Anesth Analg 2004;99:840–3.
2. Vigoda MM, Lubarsky DA. Failure to recognize loss of incoming data in an anesthesia record-keeping system may have increased medical liability. Anesth Analg 2006;102:1798–802.
3. Stonemetz J, Lagasse R. Rationale for purchasing an AIMS. In: Stonemetz J, Ruskin K, editors. Anesthesia informatics. London: Springer-Verlag; 2008. p. 7–22.
4. Stonemetz J. Market penetration of AIMS. ASA Newsl 2010;74(2):40–1.
5. EMR sophistication correlates to hospital quality data. White paper. Chicago (IL): HIMSS Analytics; 2006.
6. Egger Halbeis CB, Epstein RH, Macario A, et al. Adoption of anesthesia information management systems by academic departments in the United States. Anesth Analg 2008;107(4):1100–2.
7. Ford E, McAlearney A, Phillips M, et al. Predicting computerized physician order entry system adoption in US hospitals. Int J Med Inf 2008;77:539–45.
8. McDowell SW, Wahl R, Michelson J. Herding cats: the challenges of EMR vendor selection. J Healthc Inf Manag 2003;17(3):63–71.
9. Muravchick S. The vendor-customer relationship. In: Stonemetz J, Ruskin K, editors. Anesthesia informatics. London: Springer-Verlag; 2008. p. 23–36.
10. Epstein R. Request for information/request for proposals. In: Stonemetz J, Ruskin K, editors. Anesthesia informatics. London: Springer-Verlag; 2008. p. 37–48.

Clinical Research Using an Information System: The Multicenter Perioperative Outcomes Group

Sachin Kheterpal, MD, MBA

KEYWORDS

- Observational research • Information system
- Electronic records • Perioperative medicine

OVERVIEW

In the past decade, the increasing adoption of electronic medical records (EMRs) has created an opportunity to leverage these systems to enable clinical research.[1] Their automated, systematic approach to medical record documentation is a natural fit for research that requires structured information. An EMR can be used to enable prospective or retrospective research, using interventional or observational techniques. Increasingly, researchers are using retrospective observational data acquired from EMRs as the substrate for their clinical research into comorbidities, procedures, situations, and outcomes that have historically presented significant challenges. The use of EMRs for clinical research carries unique challenges and opportunities not encountered during classic randomized controlled trials. This article discusses the use of EMRs for observational research in perioperative medicine.

REGULATORY FRAMEWORK

Conceptually, any clinical research facilitated by an EMR is still subject to the ethical limitations placed on medical research in general. Even though EMR-based research is typically observational with no care interventions planned, the process of ethics

Department of Anesthesiology, Center for Perioperative Outcomes Research, University of Michigan Medical School, UH 1H247, Box 0048, 1500 East Medical Center Drive, Ann Arbor, MI 48109, USA
E-mail address: sachinkh@med.umich.edu

Anesthesiology Clin 29 (2011) 377–388
doi:10.1016/j.anclin.2011.06.002
1932-2275/11/$ – see front matter © 2011 Published by Elsevier Inc.

review by the appropriate local entity (eg, institutional review board, institutional research review committee) is still required. Although there is no clinical risk to a patient in the setting of a retrospective observational study, significant privacy and confidentiality risk does remain and must be mitigated through appropriate processes and technical infrastructure. The institutional review board is responsible for assessing the balance of risks to a given patient's confidentiality with potential benefits to future patients.

CONSIDERATIONS IN THE UNITED STATES

The Health Insurance Portability and Accountability Act of 1996 (HIPAA, PL 104–191) ushered in a new period of patient protections and rights. Although HIPAA addressed health care insurance availability and electronic data interchange standards, it also contains an important privacy rule that fundamentally altered the management of patient data. First, it defined a federal list of patient data elements known as protected health information (PHI) (**Table 1**).

Table 1
PHI data elements and data sets

PHI Element	Must be Removed for Exempt Data Set	Must be Removed for Limited Data Set
Names	Yes	Yes
All geographic subdivisions smaller than a state except for the initial 3 digits of a zip code if more than 20,000 people reside in that 3-digit zip code designation	Yes	No
All elements of dates (except year); and all ages more than 89 y and all elements of dates (including year) indicate such age	Yes	No
Telephone numbers	Yes	Yes
Fax numbers	Yes	Yes
Electronic mail addresses	Yes	Yes
Social security numbers	Yes	Yes
Medical record numbers	Yes	Yes
Health plan beneficiary numbers	Yes	Yes
Account numbers	Yes	Yes
Certificate/license numbers	Yes	Yes
Vehicle identifiers and serial numbers, including license plate numbers	Yes	Yes
Device identifiers and serial numbers	Yes	Yes
Web universal resource locators	Yes	Yes
Internet protocol address numbers	Yes	Yes
Biometric identifiers, including finger and voice prints	Yes	Yes
Full-face photographic images and any comparable images	Yes	Yes
Any other unique identifying number, characteristic, or code that can be interpreted back to the original patient identifier	Yes	No

Next, it established that the disclosures of these data must be preceded by explicit written patient consent to this disclosure. Because of the broad range of clinical, quality improvement, and reimbursement duties of a health care provider, the HIPAA waiver of consent signed by patients at the initiation of their outpatient, emergency department, or hospital visit is an all-encompassing document. It obviates the need for further patient consent when the data are shared within the confines of the health care legal entity and its business partners in the normal conduct of clinical and business operations. In 2009, The Health Information Technology for Economic and Clinical Health (HITECH) Act was enacted. One portion of the HITECH Act known as the Enforcement Rule significantly expands the responsibilities of entities working with PHI and explicitly provides 4 categories of financial penalties for inappropriate disclosure of PHI.

As a result of HIPAA and HITECH, using PHI does require additional legal commitments by the health care institution collecting the PHI. From the perspective of HIPAA, a data set can be defined as (1) an identifiable data set, (2) a limited data set, or (3) an exempt data set. Each data element is compared against the HIPAA PHI list (see **Table 1**). To be considered free of PHI and, therefore, exempt from HIPAA regulations, none of the PHI data elements can be present or derived from the data set. A limited data set may contain:

- Geographic subdivisions that contain fewer than 20,000 people
- Date of service (admission date, discharge date, date of death)
- Unique patient identifier that cannot be interpreted back into the original patient identifier.

An exempt data set still requires review by a local institutional review board to establish that it is exempt. Although an investigator may perceive their data to be exempt from institutional review board surveillance, it is the board's responsibility to offer this conclusion as a necessary check and balance for investigator-initiated projects.

INFORMED CONSENT

The local institutional review board may conclude one of several findings regarding informed consent for the data to be extracted from the EMR for research purposes: (1) written informed consent, (2) verbal informed consent, (3) no consent required, but opt-out capability required, (4) no consent or opt-out required. These decisions should be guided by a national oversight entity's recommendations; for example, the Office of Human Research Protection in the United States. However, local review boards may interpret these recommendations and precedent differently.

INTEGRATING COMPLEMENTARY DATA SOURCES TO CREATE A COMPREHENSIVE VIEW OF THE PATIENT

Although anesthesia information management system (AIMS) data are exceptionally detailed regarding the intraoperative episode itself, many patient data elements necessary for research may be missing. In particular, outcomes research attempting to correlate relationships between care interventions and postoperative outcomes must have a holistic view of the patient process, ranging from preoperative to postoperative care. A conceptual framework for the analysis of postoperative outcomes is shown in **Fig. 1**, based on the well-established Donabedian structure-process-outcomes framework.

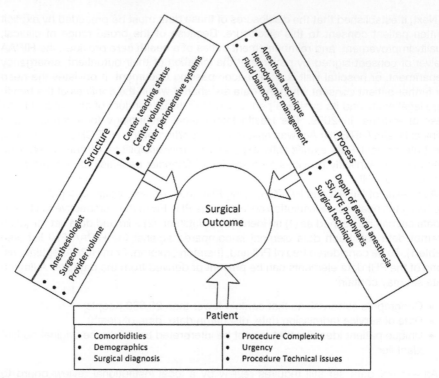

Fig. 1. Perioperative structure-process-outcomes framework.

Implicit in this analytical framework is that each component of outcome variation (structure, process, and patient) must be addressed in any analysis attempting to attribute associations to a given component. As a result, research performed using an EMR must have access to a wide variety of data elements, some of which reside in the EMR.

Identifying other data sources that contain important elements necessary for research is an essential skill.[2] Often, multiple departmental EMRs are available at a given hospital, each with unique data important for research. For example, although the AIMS may have intraoperative record data, a distinct intensive care unit EMR may be used in the postoperative care unit. Laboratory values may be stored in the hospital's enterprise EMR. Administrative data may have structured information regarding the procedures using Current Procedural Terminology (CPT) or International Classification of Diseases (ICD) codes. There are also national data sources for mortality information, such as the Social Security Death Master File for all-cause mortality or the Centers for Disease Control National Death Index for cause-of-death data. Complementary data sources that could be used for a comprehensive perioperative outcomes database are listed in **Table 2**.

In many situations, these data sources may have overlapping data elements. For example, both the blood bank database and AIMS may have data regarding blood product administration. In these situations, these data overlaps can be used to assess the quality of the data. Discordance should result in efforts to identify the optimal source of data. In some cases, the conclusion may be that the data are not usable because of missing or invalid data.

Table 2
Data sources and sample data elements

Data Source	Sample Data Elements (Among Many to be Extracted)	Interface Standards
Facility billing	Charges for ventilator days, renal replacement therapy	Yes
Laboratory	Creatinine, hemoglobin, hemoglobin A_{1c}, troponin-I, glucose	Yes
Blood bank	Units prepared, dispensed, age of units, type of unit	Yes
Pharmacy	Ordered and dispense doses of all medications: metoprolol, insulin, heparin, and so forth	Yes
Radiology	Intravenous contrast administered, interpretation of study, studies performed	Yes
Death Master File	Date of death	Yes
Surgical outcome registry	Surgical site infection, pulmonary embolus	Yes

The integration of these disparate data sources allows the creation of a comprehensive database that addresses the independent and dependent variables for most EMR-driven research projects. A conceptualization of these data is presented in **Fig. 2**.

STANDARDIZING THE FORMAT AND MAPPING OF DATA ELEMENTS

An AIMS is typically used to record preoperative history and physical information, intraoperative medication administration, procedures, interventions, ventilatory parameters, and vital signs. Unlike EMRs used in general medicine or intensive care units that depend on unstructured notes or dictations, these interventions and data elements are discrete, structured, and searchable. There are limited free-form text or prose documentation notes in the AIMS because a progress note is not the goal of the anesthesia record (**Fig. 3**). Each component of the data is stored as a distinct column in a database table, resulting in a structured EMR.

CREATING A COMMON STRUCTURE

This structured information is stored in different structures in different AIMS. In some cases, a given AIMS may be implemented differently from one site to another, resulting in the same clinical concepts (eg, arterial line access) being documented in different AIMS structures. As a result, a common structure is essential. If AIMS data are to be aggregated across sites for purposes of multicenter research, two distinct strategies are available: (1) mapping disparate structures before data transfer, or (2) mapping them after data transfer. Mapping the structures to a common data model requires significant energy at each institution. However, each institution understands its own documentation idiosyncrasies in much greater detail than any national organization. As a result, if an engaged technical and content expert are available at each site, mapping is ideally performed before data transfer. However, given the many electronic health record and clinical priorities, these resources are in short supply.[3] As a result, the mapping of disparate AIMS data structures to a single common data model may be necessary after data are transferred in variegated form. No single, common data model is right or wrong. Each has the ability to be used for certain purposes and to answer specific research or quality-improvement questions. Creating a balance between the data structure that can be completely generalized and one that is achievable remains

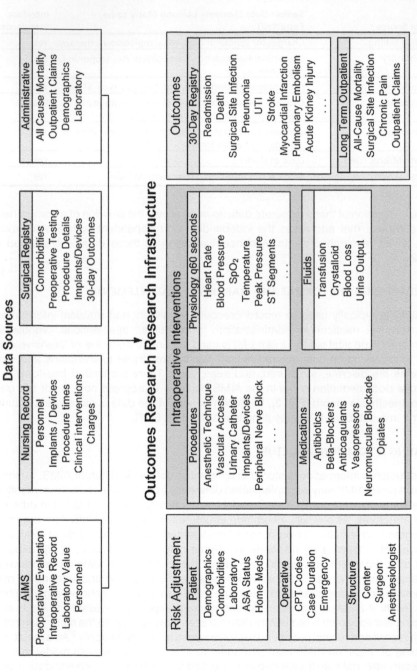

Fig. 2. Complementary data sources.

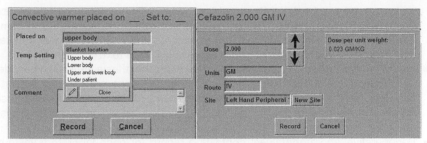

Fig. 3. Anesthesia information management system user interface showing structured data.

a challenge. For purposes of the Multicenter Perioperative Outcomes Group (http://mpog.med.umich.edu), 11 operative data structures were created:

- Patient: stores a single record for each unique patient in a given institution's database. Static information about the patient that cannot change over time is stored in this structure: race, sex, and hashed codes based on patient identifiers.
- PreoperativeCaseInfo: Multiple records for each preoperative attribute, including preoperative history and physical information; this includes American Society of Anesthesiologists (ASA) physical status, home medications, height, weight, allergies, baseline antibiotic resistance precautions, baseline vital signs (heart rate, blood pressure, Spo₂), and all comorbidities. Key elements from the surgical scheduling or nursing documentation system, such as wound classification, are also stored in this table. Because date of birth is removed from the extract to limit PHI, the patient's age on the date of the operation is stored with each operation. This age is HIPAA compliant at extremes (old or young).
- IntraoperativeCaseHeader: a single record for each operative case that summarizes basic information about the structure of care, such as surgical center type (free-standing ambulatory, ambulatory associated with acute care hospital, acute care hospital, off-site procedure area), procedure area type (off-site, main operative room, and so forth), and admission type.
- IntraoperativeMedicationDetails: many records per operation, with each dose of each medication and infusion rate change documented. Rather than free text documentation, this table is based on structured data elements, with each medication and infusion mapped to a Multicenter Perioperative Outcomes Group (MPOG) medication system number that is then referenced to RxNorm.
- IntraoperativeFluidDetails: many records per operation, with each fluid administration or output (urine, estimated blood loss) stored as a distinct record.
- IntraoperativePhysiologic: thousands of records per operation, with each vital sign (from the physiologic monitors) and device parameter (from the ventilator and anesthesia machine) recorded every 60 seconds. Structured data elements map each record to a specific clinical concept rather than free text. Where applicable, SNOMED (Systematized Nomenclature of Medicine) codes are used to define physiologic concepts.
- IntraoperativeEvents: contains dozens to hundreds of records per operation, depending on the duration of the operation. All nonpharmacologic interventions, such as intubation, placement of a forced-air warmer, nasogastric suctioning, peripheral nerve blockade, and so forth, are stored as discrete rows in this table. In addition, process times (in hospital, in room, anesthesia start, and so forth), anesthetic technique performed, airway management technique, associated

minor procedures (peripheral nerve block, arterial line, epidural), and free text documentation are stored. The amount of free text varies widely, with some AIMS and users entering minimal information via free text, whereas other sites may enter substantial portions of the record using free text.

- IntraoperativeStaffing: contains a record for each anesthesia care team provider participating during the anesthesia services. Includes the provider's role (Certified Registered Nurse Anesthetist, attending, resident), experience level for residents, and care hand offs. In addition, a surgical attending identifier is also recorded for each case.
- PerioperativeLaboratoryValues: contains a record for each laboratory value of interest within the 90 preoperative days or 365 postoperative days. Specific laboratory values are extracted from the AIMS or hospital laboratory system (hemoglobin, hematocrit, platelets, white blood cell count, prothrombin time, partial thromboplastin time, creatinine, troponin, and so forth). In addition, all intraoperative point-of-care testing, such as hemoglobin, coagulation studies, and pH, is stored.
- VenousAccess: contains a record for each venous access site used or documented during the intraoperative anesthetic.
- ProfessionalCharge: for each operative episode, the primary surgical CPT, anesthesia CPT, and operative ICD codes are stored. Anesthesiology modifiers and flat-fee CPT (for line placement, TEE interpretation, and so forth) are also stored. These elements allow structured analysis of the primary surgical procedure performed, an essential component of outcomes research risk adjustment.

MAPPING STRUCTURES TO COMMON CONCEPTS: A PREREQUISITE FOR MULTICENTER RESEARCH

Structuring data is only the first step in being able to transmit and share the data across multiple institutions. Although a medication entry may be structured, the lexicons used to describe the medication may be different or, more likely, not used at all (Fig. 3). For example, although the concept of "cefazolin" is distinct from "GM" in an AIMS database, these are simply text strings that must be mapped to consistent concepts across sites. Specifically, all physiologic parameters, medications, fluids, and outputs are stored as distinct, discrete elements in AIMS and in the MPOG data structures. For example, each vital sign observation is stored in a separate row, with a time of observation, concept identifier, value, and data source as distinct columns. In the case of a medication administration event, the name of the medication, its associated system number, dose, dose units, and route are each stored as distinct columns. Many medical lexicons are in use to describe different concepts; the lack of standardized communication may be the result of too many lexicons to choose from. Most AIMS lack tight integration with lexicons. Some specific lexicons have been approved by the Office of the National Coordinator for Healthcare Information Technology (ONC-HIT): SNOMED, RxNorm, and ICD.[4,5]

Although some vital sign concepts are already incorporated into SNOMED–Clinical terms (SNOMED-CT), there are many physiologic variables that are not. The International Organization for Terms in Anesthesiology (IOTA) effort has expanded the number of anesthesiology-specific terms in SNOMED-CT. However, ONC-HIT recently observed that there are no usable standards for a concept as simple as vital signs, despite efforts by groups such as LOINC (Logical Observation Identifiers Names and Codes) and SNOMED-CT. The ONC recommended the long-term use of the clinical document architecture (CDA). In the interim, a master list of 135 vital signs and physiologic variables across 10 different MPOG sites has been developed. For the time being, each of these variables is assigned an MPOG concept identifier.

All medications administered during surgery are stored with a medication identifier and separate columns for dose, dose units, and route. As a result, each of these concepts can be mapped to accepted lexicons such as RxNorm. A master list of intra-operative medications observed across 10 different MPOG sites has been developed. This list, now standing at 600 medications, has already been mapped to the RxNorm lexicon and the ingredient identifier for each medication is now stored in the MPOG look-up tables (**Table 3**).

In the case of combination medications, such as epidural solutions, each ingredient identifier is stored separately. RxNorm, SNOMED-CT, and IOTA terms are all publicly available, free-of-charge lexicons and are recommended by national organizations such as the Healthcare Information Technology Standards Panel and ONC.

NOVEL RECORD-LINKING TECHNOLOGIES

Although eliminating the use of PHI in EMR-based research reduces privacy risk, the absence of patient identifiers challenges traditional strategies for linking data sources. The use of PHI should be minimized, if not eliminated entirely, during the statistical analysis portion of a research project. However, creating the comprehensive research data set may require the use of PHI to integrate information across data sources. For example, the patient's medical record number would be used to merge data from disparate systems within a hospital.

However, if the data are to be transmitted outside the hospital for purposes of data sharing, it is strongly recommended that the data are transformed into a deidentified or limited data set. In either scenario, key patient identifiers usable for linking data sources are removed. However, novel record-linking technologies allow disparate data sources to be linked using unique patient codes that are not considered PHI. The use of secure hashing algorithms allows the consistent conversion of patient identifiers into alphanumeric codes that cannot be decrypted. A hashing function is a reliable, 1-way mathematical function that produces the same result when the same source string is used. As a result, the hashed identifier can be used as a unique patient key if the underlying identifiers are unique. Using hashing, patient identifiers can be removed but the resulting hashed patient keys can be sent to a centralized data center. This data center can use the patient key to collate data from disparate data sources. For

Table 3
Sample of MPOG drug identification (ID) concepts with mapping to RxNorm ingredients and drug classes

MPOG Drug ID	MPOG Drug Name	RxNorm Ingredient Code	RxNorm Drug Class
328	Recombinant factor VII	4257	BL500
19	Albuterol	435	RE102
20	Alfentanil	480	CN101
21	Alprostadil	598	HS875
23	Amikacin	641	AM300
24	Aminocaproic acid	99	BL116
377	Propofol	8782	CN203
107	Cefazolin	2180	AM115
444	Vancomycin	11124	AM900

example, institution A can send its AIMS and surgical registry data with hashed patient keys to a centralized server. Next, the centralized data center can obtain a national data source, such as the Social Security Death Master File, third party payer data, or national pharmacy fulfillment information such as RxHub. If the patient identifiers in these data are hashed using the same algorithm, patient-specific records can be linked without the use of patient identifiers. Although computationally intensive, the use of public-domain algorithms such as the National Security Agency's Secure Hashing Algorithm–256 (SHA-256) is inexpensive, and cheaper than creating proprietary distributed data networks.[6] Because no patient identifiers are communicated to the central servers, the research data set is considered a limited data set under HIPAA and Institutional Review Board purview, significantly decreasing privacy risk.

The innovative impact of this hashed identifier comparison, known as record linking, is the ability to add data sources over time without the need to recollect patient identifiers from previous data sets. As a result, if additional registries or data sources emerge, they can be linked to data that have already been collected, creating synergistic value from each incremental data source.

DATA QUALITY CONSIDERATIONS

Although EMRs allow the rapid collection of large amounts of data on a large number of patients, this capability can prove to be a hindrance because the data quality becomes increasingly laborious to assess and control. For example, a prospective, observational trial may include trained data collectors using consistent definitions for each data element. This process results in high data reliability and quality.[7] However, if an EMR is used to collect the same data element, the data quality may be high or low, depending on a variety of factors. Rather than assessing a given database as a good or bad, a more nuanced analysis that reviews specific data elements must be performed.

CLINICIAN DATA ENTRY

Although clinicians may create a more accurate medical record than administrators, the data in the EMR have variant quality based on the clinician entering the data. First, if clinicians have the perception that a specific EMR data element has significant medicolegal, reimbursement, or clinical impact, they will provide higher quality data. For example, anesthesiologists typically record an oropharyngeal disproportion assessment using the Mallampati classification system. Although the Mallampati score has been shown to have significant clinical limitations in predicting difficult intubation, it remains a core component of the anesthesiologist's physical examination. As a result, a Mallampati score entered by an anesthesiologist may have higher inter-rater reliability than if entered by a nonanesthesiologist. In general, AIMS data have reliable data for clinical elements that affect the anesthesia technique and anesthesiologist: airway examination, cardiopulmonary history, and cardiovascular medications.

Conversely, if a clinician does not perceive a given data element to affect the clinical task, it is unlikely to have high data quality. For example, although hyperlipidemia may be important to a patient's long-term cardiovascular health, anesthesiologists do not perceive it to affect the risks or options for a given anesthetic. As a result, the AIMS would be a poor source of data for hyperlipidemia.

Data consistency also varies from data element to data element. Although some concepts such as a Mallampati score may seem objective, they are subjective observations. Patient positioning, phonation, effort, and provider perception can result in variant results for this data element. For example, the reliability of a Mallampati I versus

II assessment may be low. However, there is high reliability between a Mallampati I versus IV assessment. Other data elements have high, although not perfect, data consistency. The use of insulin for diabetes management is an important prognostic data element that is recorded in many AIMS. If a clear definition is established, providers will enter these data with high consistency. The AIMS typically contain highly reliable physiologic monitoring data because they are automatically transferred from the monitor itself.[8,9]

Each data element to be used in a research project based on EMR data should be assessed for data quality before data retrieval. The clinicians who enter the data should be involved in the variable selection process to inform whether they subjectively assess the data quality to be high or low. Alternative sources of data should be considered, with special emphasis on objective sources of data. For example, a study evaluating the impact of hyperlipidemia on perioperative cardiac events should consider the value of a laboratory interface with objective cholesterol data points.

RESEARCHER REVIEW OF DATA

Theoretical data value and quality must be confirmed using data review by the primary investigator. This is a laborious, manual process that is necessary for any robust EMR-based research project. Rather than simply handing the data set off to a statistical analyst, the clinical principal investigator must review the data manually, often examining thousands of rows of data. This method is valuable for a variety of reasons. First, the investigator can subjectively assess the amount of missing data: an important element of any large database analysis. Second, the investigator observes what users are entering into the EMR, as opposed to what choices the EMR may be offering them. For example, rather than choosing from a predefined list of medications, users may be manually typing in misspelled medications. Third, the investigator can assess whether the data is a sound substrate for research. Fourth, the investigator can compare a given data element and data source with another data source to assess reliability of the data.

MULTICENTER PERIOPERATIVE OUTCOMES GROUP

The Multicenter Perioperative Outcomes Group (MPOG) is a consortium of more than 30 anesthesiology departments that use an AIMS. Founded in 2008, the group has overcome the regulatory, process, political, and technical hurdles to sharing of EMR data for research.

Currently, more than 800,000 operative records from the AIMS at each site have been extracted into a single MPOG database structure, mapped to consistent MPOG concepts, and the data have been transferred to the MPOG coordinating center, the University of Michigan. Before data transfer, patient PHI was removed from each site's data. In addition, provider identifiers (name, doctor number, pager number, user identification) were removed to decrease the risk of privacy loss for the providers involved in care. These records have also been linked to the Social Security Death Master File using blinded record linking.[9]

The MPOG members and site principal investigators possess significant observational research expertise. MPOG is focused on important patient-centric outcomes that span across the perioperative continuum. Potential projects may address health care–associated infections, perioperative myocardial infarction, acute kidney injury, stroke, airway management, and optimal anesthesia techniques. Each contributing institution has equal access to the centralized repository of data stored at the MPOG coordinating center. Research proposals are refined by a multicenter publications committee that ensures that scientifically valid analyses are performed on sound underlying observational data.

SUMMARY

Clinical research using EMR data is an emerging source of scientific progress. Although EMR data collection is perceived to require fewer resources than manual chart review, there are many specific regulatory, privacy, data quality, and technique issues unique to clinical research using EMR data.

REFERENCES

1. Stonemetz J, Schubert A. AIMS. American Society of Anesthesiologists Newsletter. 2011;75(6):10–2.
2. Kheterpal S, Woodrum DT, Tremper KK. Too much of a good thing is wonderful: observational data for perioperative research. Anesthesiology 2009;111(6): 1183–4.
3. AIMS and sharing your patient data - a resource for potential users. 2011. Available at: http://aqihq.org/cim.aspx. Accessed June 10, 2011.
4. Health Information Technology: initial set of standards, implementation specifications, and certification criteria for electronic health record technology. Final Rule. Federal Register July 28, 2010;75(144):44590–654. Print.
5. Gliklich RE, Dreyer NA, editors. Registries for Evaluating Patient Outcomes: A User's Guide. 2nd edition. (Prepared by Outcome DEcIDE Center [Outcome Sciences, Inc. d/b/a Outcome] under Contract No. HHSA290200500035I TO3.) AHRQ Publication No.10-EHC049. Rockville (MD): Agency for Healthcare Research and Quality; 2010. p. 143–67.
6. Digital signature standard. In: Department of Commerce NIoSaT, editor. Gaithersburg (MD): Federal Information Processing Standards Publication; 2009. p. 130 Available at: http://csrc.nist.gov/publications/drafts/fips180-4/Draft-FIPS180-4_Feb2011.pdf. Accessed June 22, 2011.
7. Shiloach M, Frencher SK Jr, Steeger JE, et al. Toward robust information: data quality and inter-rater reliability in the American College of Surgeons National Surgical Quality Improvement Program. J Am Coll Surg 2010;210(1):6–16.
8. Reich DL, Wood RK Jr, Mattar R, et al. Arterial blood pressure and heart rate discrepancies between handwritten and computerized anesthesia records. Anesth Analg 2000;91(3):612–6.
9. Hermansen SW, Leitzmann MF, Schatzkin A. The impact on National Death Index ascertainment of limiting submissions to Social Security Administration Death Master File matches in epidemiologic studies of mortality. Am J Epidemiol 2009; 169(7):901–8.

Real-Time Alerts and Reminders Using Information Systems

Jonathan P. Wanderer, MD, MPhil[a],*,
Warren S. Sandberg, MD, PhD[b], Jesse M. Ehrenfeld, MD, MPH[a,b]

KEYWORDS

- Anesthesia information management systems • AIMS
- Real-time alerts • Reminders • Clinical decision support

INTRODUCTION TO REAL-TIME ALERTS AND REMINDERS
Real-Time Alerts in Health Care

One of the hallmarks of modern medicine is the availability of large volumes of patient information including both physiologic measurements and laboratory data. Systems that analyze these data and report unexpected or abnormal conditions back to a clinician at or near the moment that these data are available are known as real-time alert systems. Real-time alert systems are found throughout health care and can be classified as simple or complex. Simple alerts include high-threshold or low-threshold alerts on parameters such as blood pressure and heart rate. Most modern patient monitors incorporate these alerts as audible alarms that trigger when out-of-bounds parameters are detected. Complex alerts permit the detection of data trends, the incorporation of multiple parameters, and transmission of alert conditions by means other than audible proximity. Reminders, on the other hand, serve to cue clinicians to clinical events that should occur but have not. This review focuses on real-time alerts and reminders both in and out of the operating room (OR).

Real-time alerts are expected to be most useful in clinical situations in which patient conditions are anticipated to change on a second-to-second or minute-to-minute basis. Outside the OR, the intensive care unit and emergency room are other acute care settings where physiologic conditions change on this short timeline. One of the first real-time alert systems described was a wireless personal digital assistant

The authors reported no conflicts of interest.

Financial support for this review was provided by 5T32GM007592 from the National Institute of Health as well as by department funds of the Department of Anesthesia, Critical Care, and Pain Medicine, Massachusetts General Hospital.

[a] Massachusetts General Hospital, Boston, MA, USA
[b] Vanderbilt University, 1301 Medical Center Drive, Nashville, TN 37232, USA
* Corresponding author.
E-mail address: jwanderer@partners.org

(PDA)-based system triggered by critical laboratory or vital sign data using thresholds. Parameters were set such that approximately one alert per day was generated.[1] Interestingly, and perhaps not unexpectedly, the PDA user was almost always the first clinician to become aware of the abnormality. This observation demonstrates both the effectiveness of and impetus for the further development of this technology.

Anesthesia Information Management Systems

Anesthesia information management systems (AIMS) store patient demographic information and continuously record physiologic data into a database during anesthesia care. Periodic querying of these databases and/or monitoring of incoming data allow for the implementation of real-time alerts with both simple and complex alert conditions. In addition to patient data, case details and surgical events are stored. Checking of the AIMS-generated anesthesia record allows for quality control measures to ensure completeness of documentation for billing and clinical purposes and facilitates notification of anesthetists when records are inconsistent or incomplete.

AIMS have benefits beyond enabling real-time alerts and reminders. The automated recording of patient physiologic data, for instance, has been demonstrated to be more reliable than human-recorded data. During critical situations, irrespective of provider experience and training, manual charting is frequently incomplete.[2] Automated systems are capable of keeping accurate records throughout these events and are recommended by the Anesthesia Patient Safety Foundation.[3]

The adoption of AIMS has not yet become widespread despite having this set of compelling features. According to one recent survey, only 44% of academic anesthesia departments have implemented or are committed to implementing AIMS.[4] Substantial funding is required to set up as well as maintain AIMS, which can be a prime barrier to adoption. Anesthesia departments that have AIMS have usually benefited from substantial financial support for both implementation and maintenance. Although AIMS can add value to a health care organization, they require significant customization to do so.[5] When well supported, however, AIMS can facilitate billing, research, and critical patient care functionality.

Clinical Decision Support

Overview

Information systems designed to improve clinical decision making are known as computerized clinical decision support systems (CDSS). The construction of these systems is motivated by the acknowledgment that human beings are imperfect implementers of clinical protocols and best practices with a finite ability to memorize important lists such as drug-drug interactions. The overall goal of CDSS is to improve patient care by leveraging the benefits of information technology. The use of CDSS began with the availability of computers within the clinical environment, and its effectiveness using computer-based reminders was first evaluated in 1976.[6] Not unsurprisingly, this early report notes that "it appears that the prospective reminders do reduce errors, and that many of these errors are probably due to man's limitations as a data processor rather than to correctable human deficiencies."

A recent review of CDSS found 100 published articles examining the impact of CDSS on provider performance and patient outcomes.[7] CDSS were found that support a diverse variety of medical fields, including psychiatry, medicine, surgery, and pediatrics. Decision support was provided via numerous mechanisms, including reminders or protocol presentations at time of order entry, printed reminders that were placed into patient charts, reminder pages, and automated e-mails. Performance and patient outcomes were improved in 76% of the 21 reminder-based studies, although no study showed improvements in major patient outcomes such as mortality. Most systems were designed and built by study authors (72%), and almost all were targeted at physician users (92%).

Different types of decision support

AIMS-based decision support in the OR can be grouped into 3 distinct categories: (1) managerial, (2) process of care, and (3) outcome-based decision support. Each category of decision support brings with it a varying degree of benefits, consequences, and difficulties in terms of implementation.

Managerial decision support focuses on helping providers interpret real-time data to more efficiently use the global set of resources made available to them at any particular time. This decision support includes efforts to maximize OR efficiency and throughput, decrease costs, and optimize deployment of OR personnel. Examples include the prediction of when a surgical case is likely to end through the use of live inputs, historical models, and Bayesian analysis to obtain operational efficiencies or the reassignment of postanesthesia care unit (PACU) bed request priorities when there is either an actual or impending PACU waiting list or delay to facilitate overall OR throughput. Both examples have as a goal facilitation of distinct managerial tasks such as maximizing case completion rates and minimizing off-hours OR use and overtime.

Process of care decision support focuses on allowing providers to improve adherence to clinical protocols, guidelines, and standards of care. Process of care issues are typically many times more urgent than managerial decision support concerns, and examples include efforts to ensure that prophylactic antibiotics are received within 1 hour of surgical incision, maintenance of normothermia, and glucose monitoring in patients who are at risk for hyperglycemia or hypoglycemia.

Outcome-based decision support focuses on rewarding, incentivizing, and facilitating care that leads to better patient outcomes downstream. Because the data sources that allow measurement of meaningful patient outcomes are downstream from the perioperative environment, efforts at implementing this type of decision support have been quite limited to date.

Technical considerations

One of the primary concerns of CDSS end users, and one of the important factors in determining the success of a CDSS intervention, is ergonomic management. Successful integration of CDSS into clinical workflow can result in a seamless implementation with a high impact on provider performance and/or patient outcomes, whereas poor integration can lead to frustrated clinicians and little impact. The most successful CDSS blend into the workflow rather than interrupt it; these systems "present the right information, in the right format, at the right time, without requiring special effort."[8]

Additional strategies for altering clinician behavior include education and individualized feedback, and these approaches can easily be used together. As an example, an anesthesia group set out to improve completion of quality assurance documentation, which started at a baseline completion rate of 48%.[9] Education, workflow integration, and individual performance feedback were incorporated and resulted in a stepwise improvement of completion rates (55%, 68%, and 78%, respectively). The impact of education and feedback tended to fade with time, whereas further improvement in the workflow via user interface optimization ultimately resulted in a completion rate of 94%. Studies that rely on reminders alone have also noted their impact fading with time.[10]

As noted earlier, the practice of anesthesia involves making time-critical decisions, thus alerts and reminders function most effectively when operating at the temporal resolution of seconds to minutes rather than hours to days. However, latency becomes noticeable and problematic when designing real-time interventions. Physiologic monitors obtain data at variable or clinician-specified intervals, which are then transmitted to AIMS at a predefined interval, which are in turn analyzed by decision support functions that operate on an intervention-specific interval. CDSS that depend on events documented by the user, such as case start time, are subject to additional documentation latency as well as incompleteness. The cumulative effect of these intervals needs to be carefully considered when designing CDSS.[11] AIMS typically are able to provide granularity for data on a 1-minute basis. By contrast, reliable and timely detection of critical events such as hypotension and hypoxia requires maximum sampling intervals of 36 seconds and 13 seconds, respectively.[12] Until a technical solution to the problem of latency is at hand, real-time alerts and reminders in anesthesia are able to address only a subset of clinical issues.

In addition to the problem of data latency, data reliability remains an issue. Sources of artifacts within the OR environment abound, such as misplaced pulse oximeter probes, poorly sized blood pressure cuffs, improperly aligned pressure transducers, temporarily artifact in transducer signal because of blood draws or calibration, and other issues. Ideally, erroneous signals are marked as such via AIMS by the end user before CDSS analyze these data, but, in practice, the effort required to mark every data point affected by artifact in real time is unrealistic. As a consequence, CDSS-triggered alerts and reminders must be interpreted by the clinician within the context of what is known about the reliability of the information on which the intervention is based.

Alerting functions
Several modalities of alerting or reminding clinicians have already been mentioned, specifically e-mail, pages, printed messages placed in patient charts, and on-screen reminders. On-screen reminders can be further classified as hard-stop interruptions that require management before additional work can be performed, soft-stop interrupts that can be acknowledged or delayed, as well as nonmodal notifications that do not block software interaction at all. In addition, investigative work has been performed on optimizing audible alerts, although the sheer number of OR devices using this alert functionality somewhat limits enthusiasm for introducing more sources of noise.[13] Tactile alerting functions have also been explored, although so far are not in widespread use.[14] The final frontier in anesthesia alerting technology seems to be the use of heads-up display, in which bionic anesthetists view messages beamed directly to their field of view.[15]

PROOF OF CONCEPTS IN THE PEER-REVIEWED LITERATURE
Drug Dosing Reminders

The implementation of antibiotic dosing reminders has proved popular as a CDSS task because preoperative antibiotic administration has a firm clinical basis, is frequently analyzed as a quality measure, does not require a low-latency system, and should occur within a narrow specific time frame within an anesthetic. Improvement after implementation of antibiotic reminders depends in part on preintervention compliance rates and appropriate workflow integration. Simple computer prompting, for instance, increased adherence from 20% to 58%.[16] Incorporation of antibiotic reminders within an anesthetic text task list, along with reminder e-mails stating the provider's performance relative to peers, improved timely administration from 69% to 92%.[17] The use of a visual reminder, rather than a text reminder, has also been demonstrated to improve administration practices.[18]

Drug-Drug Interactions

As much as 19% of medical errors can be attributed to complications of drug administration, such as allergic reactions and drug-drug interactions.[19] In the outpatient and inpatient setting, numerous CDSS have been deployed aimed at reducing medication errors, and, in some settings, this has resulted in a 55% reduction in error rate compared with pre-CDSS adoption. Typically, these CDSS are implemented within a computerized physician order entry system. This approach makes these safety efforts difficult to translate to the OR environment because medication administration is most often documented retrospectively, rendering drug-drug interaction detection moot in the typical perioperative workflow. However, the use of simple bar code readers and software that can facilitate recording drug doses just before administration has been shown to reduce errors.[20]

Revenue Capture

One of the key areas for the realization of the value proposition for AIMS is the facilitation of billing via automated monitoring of documentation completeness. Ensuring reimbursement for arterial line placement, for instance, is a task well suited to CDSS because it is straightforward to detect the presence of arterial line data and the absence of arterial line documentation and/or compliance. Documentation reminders delivered via e-mail and paging for one group resulted in an increase in compliance from 80% to 98%, with an estimated increase of $40,500 in annual revenue.[21] Similarly, entire anesthesia records can be checked for essential elements. The authors' group used paging reminders to reduce rates of incomplete charting from 1.31% to 0.04% and reduce time for correcting anesthesia records, increasing revenue by an estimated $400,000 per year.[22]

Cost Reduction

In addition to improving revenue capture, CDSS can also be used to reduce costs. Choosing a low-cost inhalation agent, for instance, and using low fresh gas flows (FGF) are 2 simple methods for decreasing the cost of providing an anesthetic. An individual feedback intervention performed with AIMS data but implemented with a departmental chair letter resulted in an initial decrease of 26% in FGF, which decreased over time to 19%.[23] The same study paradoxically demonstrated an unexplained and statistically significant increase in high-cost inhalation agent use, although small in effect (isoflurane use decreased from 76% to 73%).

Postoperative Nausea and Vomiting

Addressing adherence to institutional treatment guidelines for postoperative nausea and vomiting (PONV) has been another area of interest. By mandating entry of PONV risk factor data and providing an on-screen alert when PONV prophylaxis is indicated but not given, one group was able to increase compliance with guidelines from 38% to 73%.[24] After the reminder and risk factor data entry were disabled, compliance returned to preintervention baseline with an adherence rate of 37%.

Alarm Use After Cardiopulmonary Bypass

During cardiopulmonary bypass, lack of pulsatile blood flow can trigger physiologic monitor alarms, which in turn can result in practitioners turning off alarm functionality. After coming off bypass and before intervention, the rate of monitor alarm reactivation at one institution was a dismal 22%.[25] An AIMS-based alert was developed capable of detecting postbypass vital signs and notifying the provider to reactivate monitor alarms if they were disabled. The alarm reactivation rate climbed to 63% after the functionality was enabled and up to 83% after one educational session regarding the reminder. Of note, this intervention required the recording of monitor alarm status into the AIMS record, which is not always transmitted.

DISCUSSION AND FUTURE DIRECTIONS

The earlier review of the literature reveals a diverse set of successful AIMS-based CDSS interventions that have positively affected anesthesia care in a variety of areas. The experience of AIMS-based CDSS mirrors the experiences of CDSS outside the OR and is notable for 3 specific themes.

The first theme noted is that long-term success is achieved by designing an intervention that is seamlessly integrated into workflow and can be left permanently implemented without disruption. Ideally, a reminder or alert is set to trigger at an opportune time or is delivered by a mechanism that does not interrupt ongoing workflow. These mechanisms include but are not limited to paging and nonmodal reminders.

The second theme is that most successful interventions are conceived, implemented, and tracked by clinicians who are addressing appropriately selected problems. At the moment, because of latency limitations, the problem domain is restricted to those amenable to reminders that may arrive within several minutes of a triggering event, rather than within seconds. Another consideration when selecting an area to address is that a greater intervention effect is achieved by tackling a problem for which baseline behavior is far from ideal, rather than already close to it.

The third theme is that successful CDSS implementations usually include more than the simple activation of a reminder or alert. Instead, adjuvants are added such as an educational component or feedback via another communication channel. Both these types of efforts have consistently demonstrated improvements in intervention effect, although, of note, some interventions worked without the use of feedback.

Looking forward, it is clear that AIMS-based interventions will continue to be developed as additional institutions adopt AIMS technology and achieve some of the care improvements that the addition of real-time alerts and reminders can provide. Without question, these projects will continue to require substantial resources to create effective implementations because they necessitate a complete understanding of existing clinical workflow and appropriate design of interventions. Additional areas ripe for intervention will be explored, and it is likely that there will be at least a proof of concept solution for the latency issue. Although AIMS databases and/or available storage may limit monitor recording resolution to 1-minute intervals, it is feasible to develop alert technology that continuously analyzes monitor data and is also integrated with AIMS. With this development, there will be no limitation in scope to clinical problems that AIMS with CDSS can address.

SUMMARY

This article explored the adoption of real-time physiologic alerts and clinical reminder systems within the hospital environment, focused on perioperative care. As AIMS become more prevalent, use of these information systems to improve patient care, reduce costs, and enable accurate billing will become more common. Existing alert systems already function across a variety of arenas within the perioperative environment, and these systems will likely continue to diversify as health care information systems become more integrated. Successful deployment of clinical alerts and reminders requires thoughtful consideration of existing workflow and appropriately selected interventions.

REFERENCES

1. Shabot MM, LoBue M. Real-time wireless decision support alerts on a palmtop PDA. Proc Annu Symp Comput Appl Med Care 1995;(19):174-7.
2. Devitt JH, Rapanos T, Kurrek M, et al. The anesthetic record: accuracy and completeness. Can J Anaesth 1999;46(2):122-8.
3. Muravchick S, Caldwell JE, Epstein RH, et al. Anesthesia information management system implementation: a practical guide. Anesth Analg 2008;107(5): 1598-608.
4. Egger Halbeis CB, Epstein RH, Macario A, et al. Adoption of anesthesia information management systems by academic departments in the United States. Anesth Analg 2008;107(4):1323-9.
5. Egger Halbeis CB, Epstein RH. The value proposition of anesthesia information management systems. Anesthesiol Clin 2008;26(4):665-79, vi.
6. McDonald CJ. Protocol-based computer reminders, the quality of care and the non-perfectability of man. N Engl J Med 1976;295(24):1351-5.
7. Garg AX, Adhikari NK, McDonald H, et al. Effects of computerized clinical decision support systems on practitioner performance and patient outcomes: a systematic review. JAMA 2005;293(10):1223-38.
8. James BC. Making it easy to do it right. N Engl J Med 2001;345(13):991-3.
9. Vigoda MM, Gencorelli F, Lubarsky DA. Changing medical group behaviors: increasing the rate of documentation of quality assurance events using an anesthesia information system. Anesth Analg 2006;103(2):390-5.
10. Demakis JG, Beauchamp C, Cull WL, et al. Improving residents' compliance with standards of ambulatory care: results from the VA Cooperative Study on Computerized Reminders. JAMA 2000;284(11):1411-6.
11. Epstein RH, Dexter F, Ehrenfeld JM, et al. Implications of event entry latency on anesthesia information management decision support systems. Anesth Analg 2009;108(3):941-7.
12. Derrick JL, Bassin DJ. Sampling intervals to record severe hypotensive and hypoxic episodes in anesthetised patients. J Clin Monit Comput 1998;14(5): 347-51.
13. McNeer RR, Bohorquez J, Ozdamar O, et al. A new paradigm for the design of audible alarms that convey urgency information. J Clin Monit Comput 2007; 21(6):353-63.
14. Ng JY, Man JC, Fels S, et al. An evaluation of a vibro-tactile display prototype for physiological monitoring. Anesth Analg 2005;101(6):1719-24.
15. Liu D, Jenkins SA, Sanderson PM, et al. Monitoring with head-mounted displays: performance and safety in a full-scale simulator and part-task trainer. Anesth Analg 2009;109(4):1135-46.
16. St Jacques P, Sanders N, Patel N, et al. Improving timely surgical antibiotic prophylaxis redosing administration using computerized record prompts. Surg Infect (Larchmt) 2005;6(2):215-21.
17. O'Reilly M, Talsma A, VanRiper S, et al. An anesthesia information system designed to provide physician-specific feedback improves timely administration of prophylactic antibiotics. Anesth Analg 2006;103(4):908-12.
18. Wax DB, Beilin Y, Levin M, et al. The effect of an interactive visual reminder in an anesthesia information management system on timeliness of prophylactic antibiotic administration. Anesth Analg 2007;104(6):1462-6.
19. Bates DW, Cohen M, Leape LL, et al. Reducing the frequency of errors in medicine using information technology. J Am Med Inform Assoc 2001;8(4):299-308.

20. Webster CS, Mathew DJ, Merry AF. Effective labelling is difficult, but safety really does matter. Anaesthesia 2002;57:201–2.
21. Kheterpal S, Gupta R, Blum JM, et al. Electronic reminders improve procedure documentation compliance and professional fee reimbursement. Anesth Analg 2007;104(3):592–7.
22. Spring SF, Sandberg WS, Anupama S, et al. Automated documentation error detection and notification improves anesthesia billing performance. Anesthesiology 2007;106(1):157–63.
23. Body SC, Fanikos J, DePeiro D, et al. Individualized feedback of volatile agent use reduces fresh gas flow rate, but fails to favorably affect agent choice. Anesthesiology 1999;90(4):1171–5.
24. Kooij FO, Klok T, Hollmann MW, et al. Decision support increases guideline adherence for prescribing postoperative nausea and vomiting prophylaxis. Anesth Analg 2008;106(3):893–8.
25. Eden A, Pizov R, Toderis L, et al. The impact of an electronic reminder on the use of alarms after separation from cardiopulmonary bypass. Anesth Analg 2009; 108(4):1203–8.

Shortcomings and Challenges of Information System Adoption

Michael M. Vigoda, MD, MBA[a],*, Brian Rothman, MD[b],
Jeffrey A. Green, MD[c]

KEYWORDS

- Anesthesia information systems • Anesthesia informatics
- Electronic medical records

In the past decade, there has been an increase in the rate of implementation of anesthesia information management systems (AIMS) and a gradual maturation of the commercially available software.[1] More recently, as a result of the American Recovery and Reinvestment Act of 2009 ("stimulus package"), a similar pattern has been noted for enterprise-wide electronic medical record software.

Although the prospect of picking the "best" AIMS may appear overwhelming, one must recognize that this type of software requires configuration for adaptation to individual institutions. More important than the choice of software is the time spent configuring it for your needs. Examples of commercially available systems that have been in use for many years include the following:

- GE (Michigan [Ann Arbor, MI, USA])
- Picis (Mayo [Rochester, NY, USA], M.D. Anderson [Houston, TX, USA], University of Miami)

The authors have nothing to disclose.
Disclaimer: The authors are strong proponents of electronic medical records. Nonetheless, in our combined 25 years of experience using 3 different anesthesia information management systems (2 of which were purchased from vendors and 1 was developed in-house) we have experienced some of the realties that must be faced when one transitions from a paper-based to an electronic format for clinical documentation. Recognition of common challenges accompanying the implementation of an anesthesia information system is key to success.
a Center for Informatics and Perioperative Management, University of Miami Health System, University of Miami Miller School of Medicine, 1611 NW 12th Street, Miami, FL 33136, USA
b Department of Anesthesiology, Vanderbilt University Medical Center, 1301 Medical Center Drive, 4648 The Vanderbilt Clinic, Nashville, TN 37232, USA
c Department of Anesthesiology, Virginia Commonwealth University Medical Center, 1200 East Broad, West Hospital 7N-102, PO Box 980695, Richmond, VA 23298, USA
* Corresponding author.
E-mail address: mvigoda@med.miami.edu

Anesthesiology Clin 29 (2011) 397–412
doi:10.1016/j.anclin.2011.05.010
1932-2275/11/$ – see front matter © 2011 Elsevier Inc. All rights reserved.

anesthesiology.theclinics.com

- Compurecord (Mt. Sinai [New York City, NY, USA], Beth Israel-Deaconess [Boston, MA, USA])
- Docusys (Southeast Alabama Medical Center [Dothan, AL, USA], University of Pennsylvania)
- Innovian (Thomas Jefferson [Philadelphia, PA, USA], Virginia Commonwealth University [Richmond, VA, USA])
- iMDSoft (Massachusetts General Hospital [Boston, MA, USA])
- Acuitec (Vanderbilt [Nashville, TN, USA])
- Frontiers, formerly Eko (Inova Health system [Fairfax, VA, USA]).

Inevitably, no AIMS software will meet all users' needs. Although some may feel that this represents shortcomings in available products, one must recognize that the same institutional pride that typifies "that is how we do it here" implies that no product will satisfy all of one's functional requirements.

SHORTCOMINGS WITH ELECTRONIC MEDICAL RECORDS

Although there are some reports (see later in this article) of unexpected consequences that have occurred as a result of using AIMS, there is a greater body of literature pertaining to an enterprise-wide system for several reasons. First, enterprise-wide electronic medical record (EMR) users vastly outnumber AIMS users and thus there are more opportunities for potential issues. Second, enterprise-wide systems have been in place, albeit in some cases in only selected parts of the enterprise, far longer than the typical AIMS. Finally, as enterprise systems touch more types of users than AIMS, the breadth of issues is greater.

Unanticipated consequences have been reported after implementation of EMRs and range from changes in workflow and power structure, new work/more work, and persistent need for paper to far more serious concerns.[2] A study at Children's Hospital of Pittsburgh found an unexpected increased mortality in a pediatric intensive care unit after the introduction of Computerized Physician Order Entry.[3] Koppel, a sociologist, and colleagues[4,5] found that the introduction of computerized physician order entry facilitated errors when using commercially available software. Shortcomings in bar coding medication administration's design, implementation, and workflow integration can result in workarounds that can include wrong administration of medications, wrong doses, wrong times, and wrong formulations.[6] In general, these shortcomings result when paper-based workflows are maintained in an environment where electronic documentation has been implemented.

SHORTCOMINGS WITH ANESTHESIA INFORMATION MANAGEMENT SYSTEMS

Anesthesiologists, particularly those supervising other providers (ie, residents or certified registered nurse anesthetists [CRNAs]), should be aware of the time-stamping of all user-entered data, such as documentation required by the Centers for Medicare and Medicaid Services. Documenting events (or presence in the operating room) in advance of their actual occurrence necessitated a settlement by an academic practice when a claim was made regarding substandard care.[7] Other changes in workflow practices that result from the use of EMRs may be problematic as well. The ease with which users can point and click on predefined events is fairly standard in most AIMS. However, this may also lead to legible (but inaccurate) documentation where the patient is transported to the operating room (OR), monitors placed, preoxygenated, easily ventilated, and intubated during the same minute that the arterial line, central line, and transesophageal echo probe are placed.

Most AIMS have one feature universally appreciated by most anesthesiologists: automated recording of vital signs as well as data from ventilators and awareness monitors. However, although being freed of the need to manually record (and edit) these data on paper, concern about artifacts dissuades some from using AIMS and worries others about the medico-legal implications of automated recording. Most AIMS allow users to manually edit data that may create more medico-legal concerns than they solve. Wax and colleagues[8] found that 1 in 5 cases had 1 or more data points manually invalidated, although this amounted to only 0.08% of approximately 300 million automatically recorded data points. Individual attending anesthesiologists invalidated data on average in 1 of every 15 cases when working as a sole practitioner. Although a minority of invalidated values were manually appended with alternate values, data invalidation typically resulted in smoothing of the data, a common occurrence in paper-based anesthesia records as well.[9]

Reliance on automated recording has proven problematic when it was not apparent to anesthesia providers that interruption of data flow has occurred. Failure to detect a loss of incoming data when using an automated anesthesia record-keeping application weakened the defense in a malpractice claim, but spurred the vendor to develop an obvious alert to notify the user.[10]

Although clinical decision support tools offer the potential of increased patient safety, initially vendors did not offer this functionality. Now that their products are maturing, these tools are either part of the standard offering or are available for an additional expense. Although individual institutions with long-standing experience using AIMS developed in-house applets to query the AIMS database in real-time, vendors now offer a so-called "rules engine" that allows the development of rules for triggering an alert. The value of real-time alerts has been demonstrated in improving both operational efficiencies as well as clinical care.[11–13] However, when notification is triggered by real-time events (either automated data collection or user-entered data), the latency between the occurrence of the actual event and transmission to the device responsible for notification may affect the potential value of the alert.[14] Lack of time synchronization and/or back timing (antedating) of documentation may not only prevent alerts from being received, they may also result in erroneous alerts being sent. Alerts can be displayed on the OR monitor, as well as sent to mobile devices.

CHALLENGES OF MOBILE COMPUTING
Mobile Computing Added Value

The introduction of powerful mobile computing hardware allows vital information to be provided to clinicians without the need for a desktop computer. This untethering from a physical location is ideal for anesthesiologists. Often clinicians are asked to cover multiple anesthetic locations quite some distance apart, requiring them to be away from one or more locations at a time.

One such example, developed by Vanderbilt University Medical Center, is an iPhone app, VigiVU. The application works with a situational awareness program, Vigilance (Acuitec, LLC, Nashville, TN, USA). VigiVU brings vital sign data to the clinician through a mobile device, enabling proactive decision making. Older-generation personal digital assistants (PDAs), such as the Palm Treo, were found to improve communication, thereby saving clinicians time while creating opportunities for enhanced patient care.[15] The current generation of smartphones is more powerful and versatile, suggesting that additional opportunities are forthcoming.

VigiVU can receive live room video, vital signs, and notification of out-of-range vital signs. Access to laboratory values, history, and physical information is also available (**Fig. 1**). This allows clinicians to learn of evolving intraoperative events at essentially

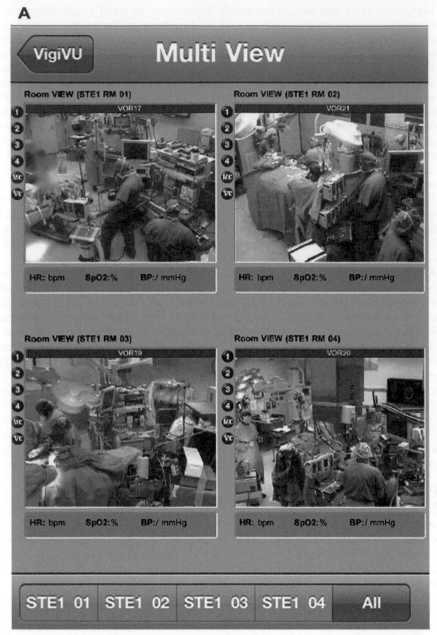

Fig. 1. Caseview screen shots of the iPhone application VigiVU: (*A*) Multiview showing 4 rooms simultaneously. (*B*) Communication panel with the room and staff signed into the case. (*C*) Focused history and physical. (*D*) Graphical vitals trends.

B

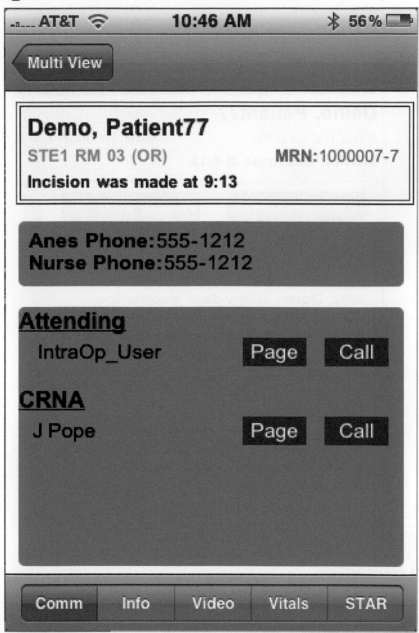

Fig. 1. (*continued*)

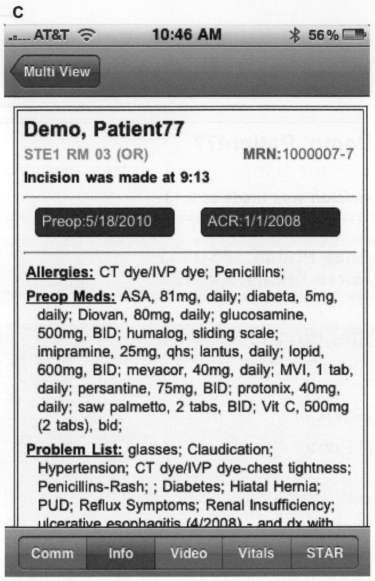

Fig. 1. (*continued*)

the same time as in-room staff (**Fig. 2**). The devices allow clinicians to directly communicate with room personnel to guide treatment either from another care area or in transit to that care location. The operating room case schedule, complete with admission, discharge, and transfer color-coding, is also available (**Fig. 3**), so that mobile technology can match clinicians' practice demands.

The Good and Bad of Situational Awareness

Situational awareness (SA) refers to "the perception of elements in the environment within a volume of time and space, the comprehension of their meaning and the

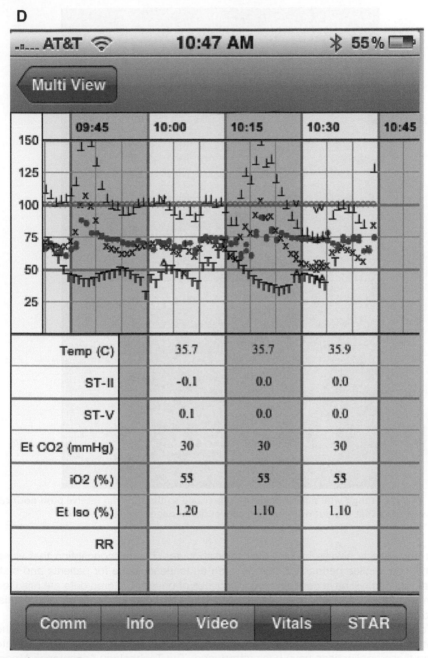

Fig. 1. (*continued*)

projection of their status in the near future."[16] The potential for proactive decision making, communication, simultaneous monitoring of separate care locations, and possibly safer care are desirable qualities of SA. Notwithstanding, there are cultural barriers to accepting such technological oversight. Providers in the room may feel

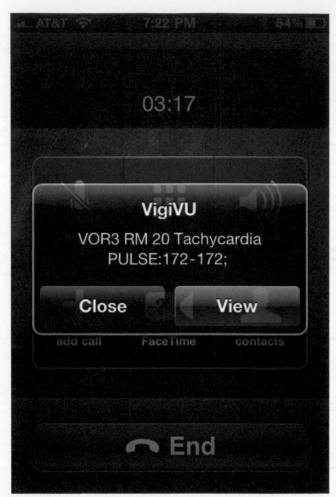

Fig. 2. Out-of-range vital signs. Rooms are subscribed so the user can receive push notifications of vitals that are out of range and conventional pages are also received.

that someone is always looking over their shoulder. The misconception that video monitoring implies permanent storage is an educational issue for patients and staff alike. Patients will have concerns regarding loss of privacy if stored data are misused or mishandled. Staff will have similar concerns compounded by fears of potential medicolegal discovery, loss of autonomy, and performance monitoring.

Educating staff about the video's intended use in a staged fashion improves the chance of acceptance.[17] The lack of user acceptance has led to a 30% failure rate when these applications have been introduced. The Technology Acceptance Model (TAM) suggests that perceived ease of use directly affects the perceived usefulness and together they best predict system use. Interestingly, technical support and training have no effect.[18]

Questionable and even inappropriate behaviors can also occur. Clinicians may feel the systems are sufficient for monitoring and present themselves in the room less often, if at all. These behaviors may diminish the benefits of the SA system. Activity

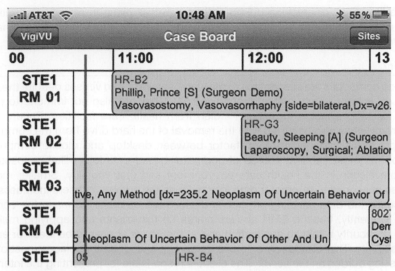

Fig. 3. Operating room case board.

logs or positioning software to review professional conduct with respect to SA system use may be necessary. The cost of staff education and remediation should not be ignored.

Mobile device safety may be a concern to some. Interactions between cell phone and pacemaker can occur. However, current devices affect pacemakers only within 10 cm and result in inhibition only. The inhibition resolves when they are distanced.[19,20]

So Much Data, So Little Time and Space

The volume of health care data continues to increase exponentially. When complex patients receive multispecialty care, data overload may lead clinicians to overlook the truly relevant data elements. Filtering and sorting patient information in real time (or near real time) is a complex task. Viewing the plethora of available data on an average-size desktop is not perfect, but large monitors increase the likelihood that clinicians will more quickly find the information they are seeking. As real estate becomes smaller, laptops show fewer data, and finding the "right" information becomes more difficult. As smaller devices (ie, smartphones) are portable but have a limited viewing area, they require device-specific software to optimally combine satisfactory ergonomics with necessary functionality.

Informational Tool or Decision-Making Medical Device?

Food and Drug Administration (FDA) regulation of medical devices is rigorous. As mobile devices become more robust, they will go beyond simply providing information and increasingly contain decision-making algorithms. This may redefine them as medical devices. Qualifying as a medical device is a costly, labor-intensive process. A limited number of companies have the resources to enter this market segment. Although the potential market size is currently in question, this class of tool continues to mature and the return on investment (ROI) may lead others to develop competing devices.

Open versus closed operating systems on the devices can become a determining factor in FDA approval. Platform stability will be crucial for these medical devices.

Device "freezing" or crashing during patient care will result in a loss of situational awareness (LSA), possibly delaying information delivery and treatment. This behavior may disqualify it from becoming a medical device.[21]

Security

Desktop computers are susceptible to malware, spyware, and viruses despite the best efforts of enterprise information technology (IT). They are also not immune to theft. Entire desktop systems have been stolen from health care facilities. Patient data compromise has also occurred with the removal of the hard drive from the computer. Laptops, as an intermediate-form factor between desktop and mobile computing, may be the most frequent source of computer-based data loss—likely because of their prevalence in the health care environment and their mobility. Smaller mobile devices may pose even greater data loss risks as the number of users increases.[22]

Security and data handling on mobile devices will be major issues in the coming years. Currently, treating EMR access points as thin-clients and applying multiple layers of security within an application and at the server appear to be ideal for enterprise security. Thin-clients rely on a client-server architecture that places most of the processing burden on the server. The client is responsible for presenting the interface to the user, and the server receives inputs and produces results. This may be ideal. Administrative and hardware costs are lower and devices are worthless to thieves because there are no data on the client.[23] The inverse relationship between security and usability must be balanced as the client interface is designed. If security enforcement places too much effort on the user to enter the program or requires frequent user authentications, application use rapidly declines, as does the frequency of SA.

Several mobile device authentication methods exist. The strongest methods ask the user to present 2 identifiers (eg, something indicating user location, something related to the user, or something the user is carrying). Incorporating this into a public key encryption and applying it to a universal health care identifier has been suggested for many years. Its implementation has not been successful because of its complexity and the massive infrastructure required. Subscriber Identity Module (SIM) cards in mobile devices have been suggested. An earlier version of this technology is not secure with insufficient key length and poor encryption. Newer Universal Subscriber Identity Module (USIM) technology offers high security but is not in widespread use.[24]

Wireless and cellular security and fidelity are also concerns. WPA2 Enterprise is currently considered the most secure. As new standards develop and are implemented, legacy mobile devices may lag with users either being denied access or being weak links in the security chain. Cellular is not an ideal option either. Old GSM signals are known to be insecure and even the current 3G is not ideal. Also, during disasters or other significant events, cellular systems are likely to fail. Physical destruction, supporting infrastructure disruption, and congestion are the primary failure categories. Physical destruction of cellular equipment leading to service failure is less likely owing to redundancies built into the system. Supporting infrastructures are based on older technologies and have less redundancy and failures are more likely. Electrical distribution, without which the cellular systems cannot function, is a prime example. Congestion from the surge in cellular demand during disasters has brought down cellular networks. September 11, 2001, saw a 92% block rate in New York City. Cellular peak loads are engineered well below the demands placed on them during disasters.[25] With LSA possible when needed most, internal wireless is likely the best option with our current technology. The infrastructure must be robust, however. With mobile practice behaviors, wireless dead spots and suboptimal node handoffs can also lead to loss of SA.[26]

At the user level, firmware modifications, such as "jailbreaking" or the ability to "side load" applications that have not been properly evaluated, may make data vulnerable. Although users can be educated regarding the risks, they can still occur. Development efforts anticipating such behaviors are necessary.

HEALTH INSURANCE PORTABILITY AND ACCOUNTABILITY ACT

Changes in privacy laws will continue to affect the security and content of mobile devices. Provider requests for patient information will be subject to a minimum necessary standard in the near future. Although many clinicians believe more information is required, compliance officers will review these devices and applications and ask specific questions regarding how the information will be used. The new rule may have some benefit, however. Ironically, providing less information (but in a contextual manner) may more easily allow delivery of vital patient information to clinicians more rapidly and effectively.

CHALLENGES OF AIMS ADOPTION

Although there appears to be an increase in AIMS adoption,[22] there are still multiple barriers to adoption. These challenges can be problematic for clinicians as well as for other stakeholders in the purchasing processes (ie, hospital administrators, IT professionals, chief financial officers, and so forth). One of the first steps to overcoming these barriers is identification of all of the stakeholders and recognition of the existing barriers. In this way, some of the obstacles to successful adoption can be reduced or avoided.

Technical Barriers

Foremost among the barriers to adoption is the technical challenge of introducing an automated and computerized process to replace a manual process that has been around for more than 50 years. Although automated recording of vital sign data has been available for a long time, it is still a process fraught with technical challenges.[27] An AIMS captures data from virtually every source in the modern operating room. However, each AIMS requires individual customization to work with the vendor-specific equipment, which varies from hospital to hospital, and not infrequently, varies from operating room to operating room within a hospital. Besides the multiparameter patient vital signs monitoring equipment, AIMS must also interface with anesthesia machines, stand-alone monitoring equipment, intravenous infusion pumps, and other miscellaneous equipment so as to capture these critical data. Each item requires an interface protocol written and tested both by the AIMS vendor and the item vendor to ensure functionality. Cooperation from vendors, who may be competitors, to develop these interfaces is frequently difficult, costly, and time consuming. However, without equipment integration, the AIMS installation may be slower than anticipated, less complete than promised, and may be less than successful. Lack of sufficient existing interfaces is a major reason for the reluctance of changing to an AIMS.[28]

To achieve the maximal benefit of the AIMS "real-time" documentation of events and data, anesthesia providers may learn a new paradigm in documentation of the care they provide. In traditional paper-based anesthesia documentation, the anesthesia provider performs patient-based tasks and interventions in real time, and then documents the results of these interventions after the fact, using milestones or cues from the care episode to approximate the actual timing of events. One of the challenges with implementation of AIMS is training users to embrace real-time (or as close to real-time as possible) documentation of events in the computer. Because the vital signs are documented automatically, there is less tedious documentation required of the anesthesia provider. Therefore, the limited number of items that must be documented can often be contemporaneous with the care delivery.

Another technical barrier to adoption is the "operating room only" focus of many AIMS systems. Increasingly, anesthesia services are being delivered outside of the traditional practice setting, including non-OR locations, such as magnetic resonance imaging, interventional radiology, and gastroenterology. Most AIMS systems have not been designed with the flexibility to be customized to meet the needs of anesthesia providers in these alternate locales. For example, most anesthesia practices provide obstetric services in the labor and delivery suite. Yet very few AIMS systems have software designed for the different provision of services to these patients. Although the standard anesthesia record can be modified to fit this area of practice, it is less than ideal for proper documentation and data collection.

Similarly, AIMS vendors have focused the design and sale of their systems on the OR practices of large academic institutions, but have not been entirely successful in selling and implementing systems in most private practices or smaller hospitals. It is in these settings where outpatient procedures of shorter duration and less complexity and even office-based procedures are conducted. In these settings, AIMS are poorly designed to meet the needs of the anesthesia practitioners and vendors may find reluctance to overcoming these technical barriers to implementation.

Many anesthesia providers are looking for a "complete perioperative solution" for implementation of an AIMS. This name is deceiving, as very few vendors offer this type of solution. Often, an AIMS product will excel in a particular area of the perioperative process, but come up short in other areas. For example, one system may have an ideal intraoperative module, but the postoperative care component may be lacking. Therefore, it is important to define the scale and scope of the AIMS implementation project and determine which areas or processes to incorporate because frequently not all will be well suited to every institution. In some cases, it may be better to install a portion of an AIMS system (ie, intraoperative record, preoperative record, or postoperative module) to prevent becoming slowed or paralyzed by the scope of the project in the quest to fully deploy all aspects of an AIMS. In this way, an installing institution can be progressing toward a complete AIMS system rather than be stalled during the installation process owing to the technical barrier of overcoming an individual AIMS module that is not perfectly suited to their needs.

Finally, another technical barrier to AIMS adoption is the configuration of the anesthesia record. AIMS vendors typically provide a standard report from the AIMS system. This standard report may or may not meet the needs of the implementing institution, or local regulations or requirements. Therefore, there may the need for additional customization of the output of the AIMS, whether digital or paper based. Also, many AIMS allow system administrators and users to create scripting or triggering of automated documentation as a means of streamlining workflow processes. Sometimes the timing or sequencing of this documentation can be disorganized and disorderly, or miss important events, leading to variability and nonstandard results. The setup and maintenance of this automated documentation can be technically challenging for the novice AIMS implementer, requiring on-site customization by the vendor or user.

Cost Barriers

The hard costs of the implementation of an AIMS include the hardware, software, interfaces, networking, storage, and any costs related to maintenance agreements or support contracts. These have been estimated to cost as much as $40,000 per workstation.[29] In addition, the start-up costs for an AIMS are often competing with other IT projects and are frequently viewed as of less value to the hospital[22] when compared with other IT priorities.

However, it is the recurring costs that may serve as a major barrier to AIMS adoption. For example, any AIMS installation must account for the cost of training of the systems' users. Every anesthesia provider needs to have some hands-on time with the AIMS software to become familiar enough with its features and functionality. The time spent during training is costly to the institution in terms of the loss of productivity from each individual anesthesia provider.

Another unrecognized cost is the initial and then ongoing support necessary to operate an AIMS. Initial support involves project management and IT analyst support for defining the scope of the project, testing of the hardware and software, and design and customization of the system. Also, there will be a requirement for the increased support that is necessary during the go-live phase of the installation. Once the system is stable and running normally, there is a cost to the 24/7 technical and reference support for the system. Often this support cannot be handled by typical IT support personnel. Whether it is because of the demanding and sterile OR environment or the real-time responsiveness required by AIMS users, these systems frequently require a dedicated AIMS support team, which must be available around the clock. In the authors' (Jeffrey A. Green) own institution (Virginia Commonwealth University), we require 1 full-time equivalent AIMS support person for roughly every 25 workstations. Because of the frequent emergent and high-acuity care delivered in an OR environment, AIMS systems frequently need to be "hot-swappable" so that there is not a costly delay in the delivery of services. This degree of immediate technical support is usually not recognized by inexperienced institutions and comes at an inflated cost. Finally, support resources are necessary for database and server support, reporting and data mining, software support, biomedical engineering, and systems administrators. After all, the true value of electronic data is the ability to analyze it. Otherwise, one is spending a lot of money for an "electronified" version of a paper record.

Last, soft costs also include the usability and efficiency of an AIMS. The easier it is for anesthesia providers to simply document the results of their interventions, the easier and less costly it will be to extract that data when needed. For example, in a well-designed AIMS, it would be simple for an anesthesia provider to document compliance statements for meeting billing and regulatory requirements, leading to better compliance with this documentation. Then, it would be easier and less costly for the institution to demonstrate its compliance and to bill for the services. Such advantages can result in significant cost savings to an institution.[30]

Cultural/Organizational Barriers

There are significant barriers within an organization that prevent easy adoption of an AIMS. In some ways, the organizational climate and the degree to which other EMR technologies have penetrated the organization will greatly determine the success of the installation. Anesthesia providers who have used other computerized systems within an organization will be more likely to adopt the system. Similarly, organizations with experience implementing other EMR technologies will be more likely willing to accept an AIMS.

Often, one of the major barriers to adoption is fear of change—a consequence of the fact that the end users will be human. Whether it is the non–computer savvy anesthesiologist who lacks basic computer skills or the efficient CRNA who is an expert at paper charting, these anesthesia providers share a fear of the unknown and unexpected consequences of an AIMS. The most common fear shared by anesthesia providers before AIMS implementation is the concern of reduction in efficiency.[31]

Universally, anesthesia providers face production pressure and the introduction of a new technology into their environment can be anxiety provoking. The fear that an AIMS will slow down workflow is a common misperception that must be overcome during an AIMS implementation. Our experience has demonstrated that after the go-live phase, AIMS users reported that it takes them less time to chart, and that they are more efficient and more accurate in their documentation.[32] These data support the often-quoted remark that once anesthesia providers have used an AIMS, they "never want to go back to paper charting."

The culture of an organization can create a barrier to AIMS implementation. Like any investment in infrastructure, there must be institutional buy-in for a project of the size and scope of an AIMS installation to succeed. Besides the initial large investment, an institution must be willing to support the AIMS system with adequate personnel and resources. The vast amounts of data and knowledge gained by an AIMS system can offer significant value to the operations of an organization. It is these data that can provide the largest return on investment for the institution.

SUMMARY

- The number of institutions implementing AIMS is increasing.
- Despite the variety of software offerings, no system will provide an "out-of-the-box" solution.
- Shortcomings in the design and implementation of EMRs (and AIMS) have been associated with unanticipated consequences, including changes in workflow. These have often resulted from the carryover of paper-based documentation practices into an electronic environment.
- Situational awareness refers to "the perception of elements in the environment along with a comprehension of their meaning and along with a projection of their status in the near future."
- The new generation of mobile devices allows providers to have situational awareness of multiple care sites simultaneously, possibly allowing for improved proactive decision making.
- Although potentially facilitating safer anesthetic supervision, technologic and cultural barriers remain.
- Security, quality of information delivery, regulatory issues, and return on investment will continue as challenges in implementing and maintaining this new technology.
- There are barriers to adoption of AIMS including technical, cost, cultural, and organizational.
- Technical barriers include lack of interfaces, lack of systems designed to handle anesthesia outside the OR, lack of customization, and the unavailability of complete perioperative systems.
- Cost barriers include hard costs at startup, soft costs for ongoing maintenance and support, and soft costs related to efficiency and productivity.
- Cultural/organizational barriers include fear of change, the variable penetrance of IT solutions in the environment, and the lack of institutional support.

REFERENCES

1. Egger Halbeis CB, Epstein RH, Macario A, et al. Adoption of anesthesia information management systems by academic departments in the United States. Anesth Analg 2008;107(4):1323–9.

2. Ash J, Sittig DF, Poon EG, et al. The extent and importance of unintended consequences related to computerized provider order entry. J Am Med Inform Assoc 2007;14(4):415–23.
3. Han YY, Carcillo JA, Venkataraman ST, et al. Unexpected increased mortality after implementation of a commercially sold computerized physician order entry system. Pediatrics 2005;116(2):1506–12.
4. Koppel R, Metlay JP, Cohen A, et al. Role of computerized physician order entry systems in facilitating medication errors. JAMA 2005;293(10):1197–203.
5. Koppel R, Leonard CE, Localio AR, et al. Identifying and quantifying medication errors: evaluation of rapidly discontinued medication orders submitted to a computerized physician order entry system. J Am Med Inform Assoc 2008;15(4):461–5.
6. Koppel R, Wetterneck T, Telles JL, et al. Workarounds to barcode medication administration systems: their occurrences, causes, and threats to patient safety. J Am Med Inform Assoc 2008;15(4):408–23.
7. Vigoda MM, Lubarsky DA. The medicolegal importance of enhancing timeliness of documentation when using an anesthesia information system and the response to automated feedback in an academic practice. Anesth Analg 2006;103(1):131–6.
8. Wax DB, Beilin Y, Hossain S, et al. Manual editing of automatically recorded data in an anesthesia information management system. Anesthesiology 2008;109(5):811–5.
9. Reich DL, Wood RK Jr, Mattar R, et al. Arterial blood pressure and heart rate discrepancies between handwritten and computerized anesthesia records. Anesth Analg 2000;91(3):612–6.
10. Vigoda MM, Lubarsky DA. Failure to recognize loss of incoming data in an anesthesia record-keeping system may have increased medical liability. Anesth Analg 2006;102(6):1798–802.
11. Epstein RH, Dexter F, Piotrowski E. Automated correction of room location errors in anesthesia information management systems. Anesth Analg 2008;107(3):965–71.
12. Dexter F, Epstein RH, Lee JD, et al. Automatic updating of times remaining in surgical cases using Bayesian analysis of historical case duration data and "instant messaging" updates from anesthesia providers. Anesth Analg 2009;108(3):929–40.
13. Wax DB, Beilin Y, Levin M, et al. The effect of an interactive visual reminder in an anesthesia information management system on timeliness of prophylactic antibiotic administration. Anesth Analg 2007;104(6):1462–6.
14. Epstein RH, Dexter F, Ehrenfeld JM, et al. Implications of event entry latency on anesthesia information management decision support systems. Anesth Analg 2009;108(3):941–7.
15. Lu YC, Xiao Y, Sears A, et al. A review and a framework of handheld computer adoption in healthcare. Int J Med Inform 2005;74(5):409–22.
16. Endsley MR. Design and evaluation for situation awareness enhancement. In Proceedings of the Human Factors Society 32nd Annual Meeting. Santa Monica (CA): Human Factors Society; 1988. p. 97–101.
17. Kim YJ, Xiao Y, Hu P, et al. Staff acceptance of video monitoring for coordination: a video system to support perioperative situation awareness. J Clin Nurs 2009;18(16):2366–71.
18. Wu JH, Wang SC, Lin LM. Mobile computing acceptance factors in the healthcare industry: a structural equation model. Int J Med Inform 2007;76(1):66–77.
19. Tandogan I, Ozin B, Bozbas H, et al. Effects of mobile telephones on the function of implantable cardioverter defibrillators. Ann Noninvasive Electrocardiol 2005;10(4):409–13.

20. Tandogan I, Temizhan A, Yetkin E, et al. The effects of mobile phones on pacemaker function. Int J Cardiol 2005;103(1):51–8.
21. McCarthy G. Situational awareness in medicine. Qual Saf Health Care 2006; 15(5):384 [author reply: 384].
22. Available at: http://www.hhs.gov/ocr/privacy/hipaa/administrative/breachnotification rule/postedbreaches.html. Accessed July 10, 2010.
23. Carden S. Thin-client medical devices. Med Device Technol 2006;17(7):30–1.
24. Sax U, Kohane I, Mandl KD. Wireless technology infrastructures for authentication of patients: PKI that rings. J Am Med Inform Assoc 2005;12(3):263–8.
25. Townsend AM, Moss ML. Telecommunication infrastructure in disasters: preparing cities for crisis communications. New York (NY): Center for Catastrophe Preparedness and Response & Robert F Wagner Graduate School of Public Service; 2005.
26. Jacques PS, France DJ, Pilla M, et al. Evaluation of a hands-free wireless communication device in the perioperative environment. Telemed J E Health 2006;12(1): 42–9.
27. Zollinger RM, Kreul JF, Schneider AJ. Man-made versus computer-generated anesthesia records. J Surg Res 1977;22(4):419–24.
28. Lawrence D. Can you feel IT coming? Though adoption of anesthesiology information systems is still low, their use is rising, and will continue as ARRA approaches. Healthc Inform 2010;27(1):14–6.
29. Ginsburg JA, Doherty RB, Ralston JF Jr, et al. Public Policy Committee of the American College of Physicians. Achieving a high-performance health care system with universal access: what the United States can learn from other countries. Ann Intern Med 2008;148(1):55–75.
30. Muravchick S, Caldwell JE, Epstein RH, et al. Anesthesia information management system implementation: a practical guide. Anesth Analg 2008;107(5): 1598–608.
31. Eden A, Grach M, Goldik Z, et al. The implementation of an anesthesia information management system. Eur J Anaesthesiol 2006;23(10):882–9.
32. Poppell CD, Green JA, Arancibia CU, et al. Comparison over time of the efficiency of an automated anesthesia record keeper as evaluated by anesthesia practitioners. Abstract presented at the Society for Technology in Anesthesia 17th Annual Meeting, Orlando, January 17, 2007.

Creating a Real Return-on-Investment for Information System Implementation: Life After HITECH

Manda Lai, MD, MBA, Sachin Kheterpal, MD, MBA*

KEYWORDS

- HITECH Act • Meaningful use
- Anesthesia information management system • AIMS
- Electronic health record

On February 17, 2009, the Health Information Technology for Economic and Clinical Health (HITECH) Act, part of the American Recovery and Reinvestment Act (ARRA) of 2009, was signed into law to encourage eligible professionals (EPs) and eligible hospitals to adopt and meaningfully use certified health information technology (HIT). Through the development of a nationwide HIT infrastructure that allows for the electronic use and exchange of information, the HITECH Act hopes to improve health care quality, safety, and efficiency, as well as to reduce health care costs and disparities around the country. To support these goals and accelerate the adoption of HIT, the ARRA authorized the Centers for Medicare and Medicaid Services (CMS) to provide monetary incentives for EPs, eligible hospitals, and critical access hospitals (CAHs) that become meaningful users of certified electronic health record (EHR) technology by 2015.

INCENTIVES FOR ELIGIBLE PROFESSIONALS

On July 13, 2010, CMS published its final rule describing the provisions governing the EHR incentive programs. EPs who can take advantage of the incentives can be any of 5 types of professionals who are legally authorized to practice under state law and be reimbursed by Medicare Fee-for-Service (FFS), Medicare Advantage (MA),

The authors have nothing to disclose.
Department of Anesthesiology, Center for Perioperative Outcomes Research, University of Michigan Medical School, UH 1H247, Box 0048, 1500 East Medical Center Drive, Ann Arbor, MI 48109, USA
* Corresponding author.
E-mail address: sachinkh@med.umich.edu

Anesthesiology Clin 29 (2011) 413–438
doi:10.1016/j.anclin.2011.05.005   anesthesiology.theclinics.com
1932-2275/11/$ – see front matter © 2011 Published by Elsevier Inc.

or Medicaid programs: a doctor of medicine or osteopathy, a doctor of dental surgery or dental medicine, a doctor of podiatric medicine, a doctor of optometry, or a chiropractor. To qualify for the incentives, the EPs must be non–hospital-based professionals who demonstrate meaningful use of EHR technology during the reporting period for the relevant payment year (ie, any calendar year beginning with 2011). To allow for some flexibility in the first payment year, CMS proposed that the reporting period be any continuous 90-day period within the first payment year; for all subsequent years, the reporting period consists of the entire year.

Beginning in 2011, and for up to 5 years, EPs in the Medicare FFS EHR incentive program are entitled to incentive payments equal to 75% of their Medicare fee schedule's allowed charges for covered professional services during each relevant payment year (**Table 1**). Under Medicare FFS, the maximum incentive payment to EPs is limited to the following: $15,000 for the EP's first payment year (or $18,000 if the EP's first payment year is 2011 or 2012), $12,000 for the second payment year, $8,000 for the third year, $4,000 for the fourth year, and $2,000 for the fifth year, for a maximum total of $44,000. However, several conditions exist: no incentive payments will be made after 2016, EPs first adopting EHR technology in 2015 or later will not receive any incentive payments, and EPs whose first payment year is 2014 will be paid starting at the $12,000 level. Moreover, payment years must be consecutive, which means that EPs have 5 years from the start of their first payment year to collect incentive payments.

To further motivate EPs to adopt EHR technology, the HITECH Act enables CMS to reduce payments to EPs who are not meaningful EHR users by 2015. Beginning in 2015, these EPs will be penalized by receiving an applicable percentage less than 100% of the Medicare fee schedule for their professional services: 99% in 2015, 98% in 2016, and 97% in 2017 and beyond. After 2017, the applicable percentage can be further decreased by 1% per year, down to no less than 95%, if the percentage of EPs who are meaningful users of EHR is found to be less than 75%. Hospital-based EPs are exempt from this payment adjustment as are EPs who qualify on a case-by-case basis for a significant hardship exception. The significant hardship exception, however, may only be granted for up to 5 years and must be renewed annually.

EPs may qualify for higher incentives through MA or Medicaid and may therefore elect to request incentive payments through these programs instead of Medicare

Table 1					
Medicare EP maximum incentive payment schedule[a]					
	EP's First Payment Year				
Year	2011	2012	2013	2014	2015 and Beyond
2011	$18,000	—	—	—	—
2012	$12,000	$18,000	—	—	—
2013	$8000	$12,000	$15,000	—	—
2014	$4000	$8000	$12,000	$12,000	—
2015	$2000	$4000	$8000	$8000	—
2016	—	$2000	$4000	$4000	—
Total	$44,000	$44,000	$39,000	$24,000	—

Abbreviation: EP, eligible professional.
[a] These amounts are increased by 10% for EPs who furnish >50% of their services in a geographic health professional shortage area (HPSA).

FFS. The MA EHR incentive program requires that a qualifying MA organization—an MA organization that is organized as a health maintenance organization (HMO)—identify the MA EPs for which it will seek EHR incentive payments. These MA EPs are individuals who are either employed by the MA organization or employed by a partner of the MA organization where they furnish at least 80% of that entity's Medicare patient services to enrollees of the MA organization. To prevent duplicate payments, these EPs must not have received any incentive payments under the Medicare FFS program. For each qualifying MA EP, the qualifying MA organization receives 75% of its reported annual MA revenue, up to the same maximum amounts as specified by Medicare FFS in **Table 1**. The penalties to qualifying MA organizations if their MA EPs are not meaningful EHR users by 2015 are the same as those under the Medicare FFS program.

EPs wishing to participate in the Medicaid EHR incentive program must meet certain patient volume thresholds over any representative 90-day period during the year. Generally, Medicaid EPs are physicians, dentists, certified nurse-midwives, nurse practitioners, or physician assistants practicing in a physician assistant–led, federally qualified health center (FQHC) or rural health clinic (RHC) who are not hospital-based and have at least 30% Medicaid or "needy individual" (ie, patients who receive medical assistance from the Children's Health Insurance Program [CHIP], patients who receive uncompensated care, or patients who receive services at no cost or reduced cost) patient volumes. Medicaid EPs who waive their rights to duplicative Medicare incentive payments may receive payments equivalent to 85% of their "net average allowable costs" for engaging in efforts to adopt, implement, or upgrade certified EHR technology in any year up to 2016. In subsequent years, these EPs must then demonstrate meaningful use of the EHR technology. The incentive payments are capped at $21,250 in the first year and $8,500 for each of 5 subsequent years (**Table 2**). Medicaid EPs may therefore receive up to 6 years of incentive payments for a total of $63,750. Unlike in the Medicare FFS program, payment years through Medicaid may be nonconsecutive.

Table 2
Medicaid EP maximum incentive payment schedule

Year	EP's First Payment Year						
	2011	2012	2013	2014	2015	2016	2017 and Beyond
2011	$21,250	—	—	—	—	—	—
2012	$8500	$21,250	—	—	—	—	—
2013	$8500	$8500	$21,250	—	—	—	—
2014	$8500	$8500	$8500	$21,250	—	—	—
2015	$8500	$8500	$8500	$8500	$21,250	—	—
2016	$8500	$8500	$8500	$8500	$8500	$21,250	—
2017	—	$8500	$8500	$8500	$8500	$8500	—
2018	—	—	$8500	$8500	$8500	$8500	—
2019	—	—	—	$8500	$8500	$8500	—
2020	—	—	—	—	$8500	$8500	—
2021	—	—	—	—	—	$8500	—
Total	$63,750	$63,750	$63,750	$63,750	$63,750	$63,750	—

Abbreviation: EP, eligible professional.

DEMONSTRATING MEANINGFUL USE OF CERTIFIED EHR TECHNOLOGY

The key to receiving incentive payments and/or to avoiding the penalties from CMS is to demonstrate "meaningful use of certified EHR technology." Consequently, the first major step to receiving these incentives is to understand and then meet the requirements of meaningful use. According to the HITECH Act, meaningful use requires (1) using certified EHR technology in a meaningful manner, (2) ensuring that the certified EHR technology allows for electronic exchange of health information to improve the quality of health care, and (3) using the certified EHR technology to report on clinical quality and other measures. To create the criteria for meaningful use, CMS and the Office of the National Coordinator (ONC) for HIT solicited input from the HIT Standards and Policy Committees, the National Committee on Vital and Health Statistics, and the public. Following these conversations, CMS decided to implement a phased approach to the requirements for meaningful use to encourage widespread EHR adoption that improves health care quality while minimizing the burdens of change on health care providers and also considering the short time frame that the HITECH Act provides for the adoption and use of certified EHR technology. As shown in **Box 1**, there will be at least 3 stages of meaningful use, each with foci that will have progressively more robust criteria.

On July 13, 2010, CMS finalized its list of Stage 1 meaningful use criteria in its final rule, structuring the list according to the 5 health outcomes policy priorities identified by the HIT Policy Committee as underlying meaningful use: (1) improve quality, safety, efficiency, and reduce health disparities; (2) engage patients and families in their health care; (3) improve care coordination; (4) improve population and public health; and (5) ensure adequate privacy and security protections for personal health information. Until CMS publishes a new list, the Stage 1 criteria will serve as the criteria that

---

Box 1
CMS meaningful use criteria foci

- Stage 1 (criteria proposed in January 2010 for 2011)
  - Electronically capture health information in a structured/coded format;
  - Use of that information to track key clinical conditions and communicate that information for care coordination purposes;
  - Implement clinical decision support tools to facilitate disease and medication management;
  - Report clinical quality measures and public health information
- Stage 2 (criteria anticipated to be updated in 2011 for 2013)
  - Expand upon the Stage 1 criteria to encourage the use of health IT for continuous quality improvement at the point of care;
  - Exchange information in the most structured format possible (eg, computerized provider order entry [CPOE], electronic transmission of diagnostic test results, such as blood tests, microbiology, urinalysis, pathology tests, radiology, and so forth)
- Stage 3 (criteria anticipated to be updated in 2013 for 2015)
  - Promote improvements in quality, safety and efficiency;
  - Focus on decision support for national high-priority conditions, patient access to self-management tools, access to comprehensive patient data;
  - Improve population health

EPs, eligible hospitals, and CAHs must meet to successfully demonstrate meaningful use starting in 2011. The list is split into 2 sets of criteria: a core set and a menu set (**Tables 3** and **4**). All of the Stage 1 criteria objectives and their associated measures in the core set and all but 5 of those in the menu set must be met to qualify for the CMS incentive payments. From the menu set, EPs, eligible hospitals, and CAHs may select the 5 criteria that they will not meet and still qualify for incentive payments. The stipulation, however, is that they must meet at least one of the population and public health criteria from the menu set.

CMS has accounted for the possibility that some criteria may not be applicable to certain types of EPs or hospitals. EPs, eligible hospitals, and CAHs are excluded from those criteria for which they neither had any patients nor sufficient actions on which to base measurement of meaningful use. For instance, EPs can be exempt from both of the population and public health criteria in the menu set if they meet the exclusion criteria for both (ie, if they neither gave any immunizations nor collected any reportable syndromic information on their patients during the EHR reporting period). Moreover, each excluded criterion reduces the number of criteria that must be satisfied by one. For example, an EP who is excluded from 3 menu criteria then needs to satisfy only 2 of them. In general, unless they can attest to meeting the exclusion criteria, EPs, eligible hospitals, and CAHs must satisfy the measure for each meaningful use objective.

One of the core meaningful use criteria requires EPs, eligible hospitals, and CAHs to report clinical quality measures to CMS. The HITECH Act gives preference to measures that are endorsed by the National Quality Forum (NQF), including those that were previously selected for the Physician Quality Reporting Initiative (PQRI) program. For Stage 1, CMS decided to require only those NQF-endorsed, clinical quality measures whose numerators, denominators, and exclusions can be automatically calculated using certified EHR technology. CMS also limited the measures to those for which electronic specifications are currently available. The list of clinical quality measures is divided into 2 groups: a core group and a specialty group (**Tables 5** and **6**). EPs are required to report on all 3 measures in the core group as well as 3 measures of their choice from the 38 listed in the specialty group. EPs simply report the numerators, denominators, and/or exclusions for each of the measures once a year, and are not required to meet any specific thresholds for these fields. If any of the denominators are 0 for the core measures then the EP is required to report on up to 3 of the alternate core measures. If all 6 core and alternate core measures do not apply to the EP's scope of practice or patient population, then the EP simply reports zeros for the denominators of each of the inapplicable measures. However, the EP is still required to report on 3 measures from the specialty group. Only EPs who attest that all of their clinical quality measures have a denominator of 0 are exempt from reporting any.

In 2011, reporting on meaningful use, including clinical quality reporting, will occur through attestation, because CMS does not believe that it will have the capacity to accept information electronically by then. In 2012, or in whatever year CMS develops the necessary capacity to accept information electronically, EPs, eligible hospitals, and CAHs will be required to submit this information electronically using their certified EHR technology and attest to the accuracy and completeness of the values submitted. Beyond meaningful use, qualification for the CMS incentive payments requires the use of certified EHR technology. For EPs, at least 50% of their practice must occur at locations equipped with certified EHR technology. On July 13, 2010, the ONC published its final rule on the standards, implementation specifications, and certification criteria for the EHR technology that EPs, eligible hospitals, and

Table 3
CMS stage 1 meaningful use criteria for EPs, eligible hospitals and CAHs: core set

Health Outcomes Policy Priority	Objective		Measure	Exclusion
	EPs	Eligible Hospitals and CAHs		
Improve quality, safety, efficiency, and reduce health disparities	1. Use CPOE for medication orders directly entered by any licensed health care professional who can enter orders into the medical record per state, local, and professional guidelines		More than 30% of all unique patients with at least one medication in their medication list seen by the EP or admitted to the eligible hospital's or CAH's inpatient or emergency department (POS 21 or 23) during the EHR reporting period have at least one medication order entered using CPOE	EPs who write fewer than 100 prescriptions during the EHR reporting period; None for eligible hospitals and CAHs
	2. Implement drug-drug and drug-allergy interaction checks		The EP, eligible hospital, or CAH has enabled this functionality for the entire EHR reporting period	None
	3. Generate and transmit permissible prescriptions electronically (eRx)		More than 40% of all permissible prescriptions written by the EP are t ransmitted electronically using certified EHR technology	EPs who write fewer than 100 prescriptions during the EHR reporting period
	4. Record the following demographics: (A) Preferred language, (B) Gender, (C) Race, (D) Ethnicity, (E) Date of birth	Record the following demographics: (A) Preferred language, (B) Gender, (C) Race, (D) Ethnicity, (E) Date of birth, (F) Date and preliminary cause of death in the event of mortality in the eligible hospital or CAH	More than 50% of all unique patients seen by the EP or admitted to an eligible hospital's or CAH's inpatient or emergency department (POS 21 or 23) have demographics recorded as structured data	None

5. Maintain an up-to-date problem list of current and active diagnoses	More than 80% of all unique patients seen by the EP or admitted to the eligible hospital's or CAH's inpatient or emergency department (POS 21 or 23) have at least one entry or an indication that no problems are known for the patient recorded as structured data	None
6. Maintain active medication list	More than 80% of all unique patients seen by the EP or admitted to the eligible hospital's or CAH's inpatient or emergency department (POS 21 or 23) have at least one entry (or an indication that the patient is not currently prescribed any medication) recorded as structured data	None
7. Maintain active medication allergy list	More than 80% of all unique patients seen by the EP or admitted to the eligible hospital's or CAH's inpatient or emergency department (POS 21 or 23) have at least one entry (or an indication that the patient has no known medication allergies) recorded as structured data	None

(continued on next page)

Table 3
(continued)

Health Outcomes Policy Priority	Objective		Measure	Exclusion
	EPs	Eligible Hospitals and CAHs		
		8. Record and chart changes in vital signs: (1) Height, (2) Weight, (3) Blood pressure, (4) Calculate and display the body mass index (BMI), (5) Plot and display growth charts for children 2 to 20 years old, including BMI	For more than 50% of all unique patients age 2 years or older seen by the EP or admitted to the eligible hospital's or CAH's inpatient or emergency department (POS 21 or 23), height, weight, and blood pressure are recorded as structured data	EPs who do not see patients 2 years old or older. EPs who believe that all 3 vital signs of height, weight, and blood pressure have no relevance to their scope of practice can attest and be excluded. None for eligible hospitals or CAHs
		9. Record smoking status for patients 13 years old or older	More than 50% of all unique patients age 13 years or older seen by the EP or admitted to the eligible hospital's or CAH's inpatient or emergency department (POS 21 or 23) have smoking status recorded as structured data	EPs, eligible hospitals, or CAHs who do not see patients 13 years or older
	10. Implement one clinical decision support rule relevant to specialty or high clinical priority along with the ability to track compliance with that rule	Implement one clinical decision support rule related to a high-priority hospital condition along with the ability to track compliance with that rule	Implement one clinical decision support rule	None
	11. Report ambulatory clinical quality measures to CMS or, in the case of Medicaid EPs, the states	Report hospital clinical quality measures to CMS or, in the case of Medicaid-eligible hospitals, the states	For 2011, provide aggregate numerator, denominator, and exclusions through attestation. For 2012, electronically submit the clinical quality measures	None

Category	Objective	Measure	Exclusion
Engage patients and families in their health care	12. Provide patients with an electronic copy of their health information (including diagnostic test results, problem list, medication lists, medication allergies) upon request	More than 50% of all patients of the EP or the inpatient or emergency departments of the eligible hospital or CAH (POS 21 or 23) who request an electronic copy of their health information are provided it within 3 business days	EPs, eligible hospitals, or CAHs that do not have any requests from patients or their agents for an electronic copy of patient health information during the EHR reporting period
	13. Provide patients with an electronic copy of their discharge instructions at time of discharge, upon request	More than 50% of all patients who are discharged from an eligible hospital's or CAH's inpatient department or emergency department (POS 21 or 23) and who request an electronic copy of their discharge instructions are provided with it	Eligible hospitals or CAHs that do not have any requests from patients or their agents for an electronic copy of their discharge instructions during the EHR reporting period
	14. Provide clinical summaries for patients for each office visit	Clinical summaries provided to patients for more than 50% of all office visits within 3 business days	EPs who have no office visits during the EHR reporting period
Improve care coordination	15. Capability to exchange key clinical information (for example, problem list, medication list, medication allergies, diagnostic test results), among providers of care and patient-authorized entities electronically	Capability to exchange key clinical information (for example, discharge summary, procedures, problem list, medication list, medication allergies, diagnostic test results) among providers of care and patient-authorized entities electronically	Perform at least one test of certified EHR technology's capacity to electronically exchange key clinical information	None
Ensure adequate privacy and security protections for personal health information	16. Protect electronic health information created or maintained by the certified EHR technology through the implementation of appropriate technical capabilities	Conduct or review a security risk analysis and implement security updates as necessary and correct identified security deficiencies as part of its risk management process	None

Abbreviations: CAH, critical access hospital; CMS, Centers for Medicare and Medicaid Services; CPOE, computerized provider order entry; EHR, electronic health record; EP, eligible professional; POS, place of service.

Table 4
CMS stage 1 meaningful use criteria for EPs, Eligible hospitals and CAHs: menu set

Health Outcomes Policy Priority	Objective		Measure	Exclusion
	EPs	Eligible Hospitals and CAHs		
Improve quality, safety, efficiency, and reduce health disparities	1. Implement drug-formulary checks		The EP, eligible hospital, or CAH has enabled this functionality and has access to at least one internal or external drug formulary for the entire EHR reporting period	EPs who write fewer than 100 prescriptions during the EHR reporting period; None for eligible hospitals and CAHs
	2.	Record advance directives for patients 65 years old or older	More than 50% of all unique patients 65 years old or older admitted to the eligible hospital's or CAH's inpatient department (POS 21) have an indication of an advance directive status recorded	Eligible hospitals or CAHs that do not admit patients 65 years old or older during the EHR reporting period
	3. Incorporate clinical lab-test results into certified EHR technology as structured data		More than 40% of all clinical lab tests results ordered by the EP or by an authorized provider of the eligible hospital or CAH for patients admitted to its inpatient or emergency department (POS 21 or 23) during the EHR reporting period whose results are either in a positive/ negative or numerical format are incorporated in certified EHR technology as structured data	EPs who do not order lab tests whose results are either in a positive/ negative or numeric format during the EHR reporting period. None for eligible hospitals or CAHs
			Generate at least one report listing patients of the EP,	None

	Objective	Measure	Exclusion
	4. Generate lists of patients by specific conditions to use for quality improvement, reduction of disparities, research and outreach[a]	eligible hospital or CAH with a specific condition	
	5. Send reminders to patients per patient preference for preventive/follow-up care	More than 20% of all unique patients 65 years or older or 5 years old or younger were sent an appropriate reminder during the EHR reporting period	EPs who do not have any patients 65 years old or older or 5 years old or younger with records maintained using certified EHR technology
Engage patients and families in their health care	6. Provide patients with timely electronic access to their health information (including lab results, medication problem list, medication lists, medication allergies) within 4 business days of the information being available to the EP	More than 10% of all unique patients seen by the EP are provided timely (available to the patient within 4 business days of being updated in the certified EHR technology) electronic access to their health information subject to the EP's discretion to withhold certain information	EPs that neither order nor create any of the information listed during the EHR reporting period
	7. Use certified EHR technology to identify patient-specific education resources and provide those resources to the patient if appropriate	More than 10% of all unique patients seen by the EP or admitted to the eligible hospital's or CAH's inpatient or emergency department (POS 21 or 23) are provided patient-specific education resources	None

(continued on next page)

Table 4
(continued)

Health Outcomes Policy Priority	Objective		Measure	Exclusion
	EPs	Eligible Hospitals and CAHs		
Improve care coordination		8. The EP, eligible hospital or CAH who receives a patient from another setting of care or provider of care or believes an encounter is relevant should perform medication reconciliation	The EP, eligible hospital or CAH performs medication reconciliation for more than 50% of transitions of care in which the patient is transitioned into the care of the EP or admitted to the eligible hospital's or CAH's inpatient or emergency department (POS 21 or 23)	EPs who were not on the receiving end of any transitions of care during the EHR reporting period. None for eligible hospitals or CAHs
		9. The EP, eligible hospital, or CAH who transitions their patient to another setting of care or provider of care should provide summary of care record for each transition of care or referral	The EP, eligible hospital, or CAH who transitions or refers their patient to another setting of care or provider of care provides a summary of care record for more than 50% of transitions of care and referrals	EPs who do not transfer a patient to another setting or refer a patient to another provider during the EHR reporting period. None for eligible hospitals or CAHs
Improve population and public health		10. Capability to submit electronic data to immunization registries or Immunization Information Systems and actual submission in accordance with applicable law and practice[a]	Performed at least one test of certified EHR technology's capacity to submit electronic data to immunization registries and follow-up submission if the test is successful (unless none of the immunization registries to which the EP, eligible hospital or CAH submits	EPs, eligible hospitals, and CAHs that have not given any immunizations during the EHR reporting period or where no immunization registry has the capacity to receive the information electronically. EPs in a group setting using identical certified EHR technology would need

11.	Capability to submit electronic data on reportable (as required by State or local law) lab results to public health agencies and actual submission in accordance with applicable law and practice[a]	Performed at least one test of certified EHR technology's capacity to provide electronic submission of reportable lab results to public health agencies and follow-up submission if the test is successful (unless none of the public health agencies to which the eligible hospital or CAH submits such information have the capacity to receive the information electronically)	onlyto conduct a single test, not one test per EP No public health agency to which the eligible hospital or CAH submits such information has the capacity to receive the information electronically
12.	Capability to submit electronic syndromic surveillance data to public health agencies and actual submission in accordance with applicable law and practice[a]	Performed at least one test of certified EHR technology's capacity to provide electronic syndromic surveillance data to public health agencies and follow-up submission if the test is successful (unless none of the public health agencies to which the EP, eligible hospital or CAH submits such information have the capacity to receive the information electronically)	EPs who do not collect any reportable syndromic information on their patients during the EHR reporting period or do not submit such information to any public health agency that has the capacity to receive the information electronically

Abbreviations: CAH, critical access hospital; EHR, electronic health record; EP, eligible professional.

[a] In the Medicaid EHR incentive program for Stage 1, states may tailor these meaningful use definitions as they pertain to public health objectives and data registries.

Table 5
Core and alternate core clinical quality measures

	Title	Description	NQF Measure Number	PQRI Implementation Number
Core measures	Adult weight screening and follow-up	Percentage of patients aged 18 years and older with a calculated BMI in the past 6 months or during the current visit documented in the medical record AND if the most recent BMI is outside parameters, a follow-up plan is documented	NQF 0421	PQRI 128
	Hypertension: blood pressure measurement	Percentage of patient visits for patients aged 18 years and older with a diagnosis of hypertension who have been seen for at least 2 office visits, with blood pressure (BP) recorded	NQF 0013	
	Preventive care and screening measure pair: a. Tobacco use assessment, b. Tobacco cessation intervention	a. Percentage of patients aged 18 years and older who have been seen for at least 2 office visits who were queried about tobacco use one or more times within 24 months, b. Percentage of patients aged 18 years and older identified as tobacco users within the past 24 months and have been seen for at least 2 office visits, who received cessation intervention	NQF 0028	
Alternate core measures	Preventive care and screening: influenza immunization for patients ≥50 years old	Percentage of patients aged 50 years and older who received an influenza immunization during the flu season (September through February)	NQF 0041	PQRI 110
	Weight assessment and counseling for children and adolescents	Percentage of patients 2–17 years of age who had an outpatient visit with a Primary Care Physician (PCP) or OB/GYN and who had evidence of BMI percentile documentation, counseling for nutrition and counseling for physical activity during the measurement year	NQF 0024	
	Childhood immunization status	Percentage of children 2 years of age who had 4 diphtheria, tetanus, and acellular pertussis (DTaP); 3 polio (IPV); 1 measles, mumps, and rubella (MMR); 2 H influenza type B (HiB); 3 hepatitis B (Hep B); 1 chicken pox (VZV); 4 pneumococcal conjugate (PCV); 2 hepatitis A (Hep A); 2 or 3 rotavirus (RV); and 2 influenza (flu) vaccines by their second birthday. The measure calculates a rate for each vaccine and 9 separate combination rates	NQF 0038	

Abbreviations: BMI, body mass index; NQF, National Quality Forum; OB/GYN, obstetrician/gynecologist; PQRI, Physician Quality Reporting Initiative.

CAHs can use to achieve meaningful use. In essence, the ONC final rule specifies the minimum capabilities that certified EHR technology must include to help EPs, eligible hospitals, and CAHs meet their meaningful use requirements. An additional certification criterion is automated measure calculation: certified EHR technology must have the capability to electronically record the numerator and denominator for each meaningful use objective with a percentage-based measure. On the other hand, certified EHR technology does not need to provide results for meaningful use criteria whose measures simply require a yes or no for attestation. EPs, eligible hospitals, and CAHs can satisfy the requirement of using certified EHR technology by using either a combination of EHR modules—EHR services and/or components that meet at least one certification criterion—or a complete EHR system that they test and certify as meeting all applicable certification criteria established by the ONC.

HOSPITAL-BASED EPs

The HITECH Act specifies that hospital-based EPs are not eligible for the CMS incentive payments and are also exempt from the downward payment adjustment penalties for not being meaningful EHR users by 2015. Examples of hospital-based EPs provided in the HITECH Act include pathologists, anesthesiologists, and emergency physicians, ie, "those physicians who furnish substantially all of their professional services during the relevant EHR reporting period in a hospital setting (whether inpatient or outpatient) through the use of the facilities and equipment of the hospital, including the hospital's qualified EHRs." Consequently, CMS initially proposed to consider EPs as hospital-based if they provide 90% of their services in inpatient, outpatient, or a combination of inpatient and outpatient hospital settings. To determine if an EP meets the 90% threshold, CMS decided that it would use the place of service (POS) codes that the EP reports on his or her physician claims forms. In April 2010, however, the Continuing Extension Act of 2010 changed the definition of hospital-based EPs to include only those who work in an inpatient or emergency room setting. Subsequently, CMS changed its hospital-based definition to include only those EPs who bill 90% of their POS codes as either 21 (Inpatient Hospital) or 23 (Emergency Room, Hospital).

IMPLICATIONS FOR ANESTHESIOLOGISTS
Scenario 1

You are an intensivist who specializes in taking care of critically ill patients in the intensive care unit. You use the hospital's EHR technology on a regular basis to input patient notes, view patient vitals and lab results, and order medications. Because you see only inpatients, 100% of your patients are billed as POS code 21, so you are considered (rightfully so in our opinion) to be hospital-based. Consequently, you are ineligible for any of the CMS incentive payments but are also exempt from any of the penalties. This makes sense, as all of the equipment, medications, and EHR technology that you use were purchased by the hospital anyway.

Scenario 2

You are a chronic pain specialist who performs facet and medial branch blocks in your own outpatient clinic. You have been thinking about going paperless for a while now; after the HITECH Act passed, you think it is the perfect time to purchase and implement a certified, ambulatory information management system. You select one that enables you to meet all of the meaningful use criteria and begin using it in 2012. Because you have adopted and then meaningfully used your certified EHR technology

Table 6
Specialty clinical quality measures

Title	Description	NQF Measure Number	PQRI Implementation Number
Diabetes: hemoglobin a1c poor control	Percentage of patients 18–75 years of age with diabetes (type 1 or type 2) who had hemoglobin A1c >9.0%	NQF 0059	PQRI 1
Diabetes: low-density lipoprotein (ldl) management and control	Percentage of patients 18–75 years of age with diabetes (type 1 or type 2) who had LDL-C <100 mg/dL	NQF 0064	PQRI 2
Diabetes: blood pressure management	Percentage of patients 18–75 years of age with diabetes (type 1 or type 2) who had blood pressure <140/90 mm Hg	NQF 0061	PQRI 3
Heart failure (HF): angiotensin-converting enzyme (ACE) inhibitor or angiotensin receptor blocker (ARB) therapy for left ventricular systolic dysfunction (LVSD)	Percentage of patients aged 18 years and older with a diagnosis of heart failure and LVSD (LVEF <40%) who were prescribed ACE inhibitor or ARB therapy	NQF 0081	PQRI 5
Coronary artery disease (CAD): beta-blocker therapy for CAD patients with prior myocardial infarction (MI)	Percentage of patients aged 18 years and older with a diagnosis of CAD and prior MI who were prescribed beta-blocker therapy	NQF 0070	PQRI 7
Pneumonia vaccination status for older adults	Percentage of patients 65 years of age and older who have ever received a pneumococcal vaccine	NQF 0043	PQRI 111
Breast cancer screening	Percentage of women 40–69 years of age who had a mammogram to screen for breast cancer	NQF 0031	PQRI 112
Colorectal cancer screening	Percentage of adults 50–75 years of age who had appropriate screening for colorectal cancer	NQF 0034	PQRI 113
Coronary artery disease (cad): oral antiplatelet therapy prescribed for patients with CAD	Percentage of patients aged 18 years and older with a diagnosis of CAD who were prescribed oral antiplatelet therapy	NQF 0067	PQRI 6
Heart failure (HF): beta-blocker therapy for left ventricular systolic dysfunction (LVSD)	Percentage of patients aged 18 years and older with a diagnosis of heart failure who also have LVSD (LVEF <40%) and who were prescribed betablocker therapy	NQF 0083	PQRI 8

Measure	Description	NQF	PQRI
Anti-depressant medication management: (a) effective acute phase treatment, (b) effective continuation phase treatment	Percentage of patients 18 years of age and older who were diagnosed with a new episode of major depression, treated with antidepressant medication, and who remained on an antidepressant medication treatment	NQF 0105	PQRI 9
Primary open angle glaucoma (POAG): optic nerve evaluation	Percentage of patients aged 18 years and older with a diagnosis of POAG who have been seen for at least 2 office visits who have an optic nerve head evaluation during 1 or more office visits within 12 months	NQF 0086	PQRI 12
Diabetic retinopathy: documentation of presence or absence of macular edema and level of severity of retinopathy	Percentage of patients aged 18 years and older with a diagnosis of diabetic retinopathy who had a dilated macular or fundus examination performed that included documentation of the level of severity of retinopathy and the presence or absence of macular edema during 1 or more office visits within 12 months	NQF 0088	PQRI 18
Diabetic retinopathy: communication with the physician managing ongoing diabetes care	Percentage of patients aged 18 years and older with a diagnosis of diabetic retinopathy who had a dilated macular or fundus examination performed with documented communication to the physician who manages the ongoing care of the patient with diabetes mellitus regarding the findings of the macular or fundus examination at least once within 12 months	NQF 0089	PQRI 19
Asthma pharmacologic therapy	Percentage of patients aged 5 through 40 years with a diagnosis of persistent asthma who were prescribed either the mild, moderate, or severe preferred long-term control medication (inhaled corticosteroid) or an acceptable alternative treatment	NQF 0047	PQRI 53
Asthma assessment	Percentage of patients aged 5 through 40 years with a diagnosis of asthma and who have been seen for at least 2 office visits, who were evaluated during at least 1 office visit within 12 months for the frequency (numeric) of daytime and nocturnal asthma symptoms	NQF 0001	PQRI 64
Appropriate testing for children with pharyngitis	Percentage of children 2–18 years of age who were diagnosed with pharyngitis, dispensed an antibiotic and received a group A streptococcus (strep) test for the episode	NQF 0002	PQRI 66

(continued on next page)

Table 6
(continued)

Title	Description	NQF Measure Number	PQRI Implementation Number
Oncology breast cancer: hormonal therapy for stage IC-IIIC estrogen receptor/progesterone receptor (ER/PR) positive breast cancer	Percentage of female patients aged 18 years and older with Stage IC through IIIC, ER or PR positive breast cancer who were prescribed tamoxifen or aromatase inhibitor (AI) during the 12-month reporting period	NQF 0387	PQRI 71
Oncology colon cancer: chemotherapy for stage III colon cancer patients	Percentage of patients aged 18 years and older with Stage IIIA through IIIC colon cancer who are referred for adjuvant chemotherapy, prescribed adjuvant chemotherapy, or have previously received adjuvant chemotherapy within the 12-month reporting period	NQF 0385	PQRI 72
Prostate cancer: avoidance of overuse of bone scan for staging low-risk prostate cancer patients	Percentage of patients, regardless of age, with a diagnosis of prostate cancer at low risk of recurrence receiving interstitial prostate brachytherapy, OR external beam radiotherapy to the prostate, OR radical prostatectomy, OR cryotherapy who did not have a bone scan performed at any time since diagnosis of prostate cancer	NQF 0389	PQRI 102
Smoking and tobacco use cessation, medical assistance: a. advising smokers and tobacco users to quit, b. discussing smoking and tobacco use cessation medications, c. discussing smoking and tobacco use cessation strategies	Percentage of patients 18 years of age and older who were current smokers or tobacco users, who were seen by a practitioner during the measurement year and who received advice to quit smoking or tobacco use or whose practitioner recommended or discussed smoking or tobacco use cessation medications, methods or strategies	NQF 0027	PQRI 115
Diabetes: eye exam	Percentage of patients 18–75 years of age with diabetes (type 1 or type 2) who had a retinal or dilated eye examination or a negative retinal examination (no evidence of retinopathy) by an eye care professional	NQF 0055	PQRI 117
Diabetes: urine screening	Percentage of patients 18–75 years of age with diabetes (type 1 or type 2) who had a nephropathy screening test or evidence of nephropathy	NQF 0062	PQRI 119
Diabetes: foot exam	Percentage of patients aged 18–75 years with diabetes (type 1 or type 2) who had a foot examination (visual inspection, sensory examination with monofilament, or pulse examination)	NQF 0056	PQRI 163

Coronary artery disease (CAD): drug therapy for lowering LDL-cholesterol	Percentage of patients aged 18 years and older with a diagnosis of CAD who were prescribed a lipid-lowering therapy (based on current ACC/AHA guidelines)	NQF 0074 · PQRI 197
Heart failure (HF): warfarin therapy patients with atrial fibrillation	Percentage of all patients aged 18 years and older with a diagnosis of heart failure and paroxysmal or chronic atrial fibrillation who were prescribed warfarin therapy	NQF 0084 · PQRI 200
Ischemic vascular disease (IVD): blood pressure management	Percentage of patients 18 years of age and older who were discharged alive for acute myocardial infarction (AMI), coronary artery bypass graft (CABG) or percutaneous transluminal coronary angioplasty (PTCA) from January 1–November 1 of the year before the measurement year, or who had a diagnosis of ischemic vascular disease (IVD) during the measurement year and the year before the measurement year and whose recent blood pressure is in control (<140/90 mm Hg)	NQF 0073 · PQRI 201
Ischemic vascular disease (IVD): use of aspirin or another antithrombotic	Percentage of patients 18 years of age and older who were discharged alive for acute myocardial infarction (AMI), coronary artery bypass graft (CABG) or percutaneous transluminal coronary angioplasty (PTCA) from January 1–November 1 of the year before the measurement year, or who had a diagnosis of ischemic vascular disease (IVD) during the measurement year and the year before the measurement year and who had documentation of use of aspirin or another antithrombotic during the measurement year	NQF 0068 · PQRI 204
Initiation and engagement of alcohol and other drug dependence treatment: (a) initiation, (b) engagement	Percentage of adolescent and adult patients with a new episode of alcohol and other drug (AOD) dependence who initiate treatment through an inpatient AOD admission, outpatient visit, intensive outpatient encounter or partial hospitalization within 14 days of the diagnosis and who initiated treatment and who had 2 or more additional services with an AOD diagnosis within 30 days of the initiation visit	NQF 0004
Prenatal care: screening for human immunodeficiency virus (HIV)	Percentage of patients, regardless of age, who gave birth during a 12-month period who were screened for HIV infection during the first or second prenatal care visit	NQF 0012

(continued on next page)

Table 6
(continued)

Title	Description	NQF Measure Number	PQRI Implementation Number
Prenatal care: Anti-D immune globulin	Percentage of D (Rh) negative, unsensitized patients, regardless of age, who gave birth during a 12-month period who received anti-D immune globulin at 26–30 weeks gestation	NQF 0014	
Controlling high blood pressure	Percentage of patients 18–85 years of age who had a diagnosis of hypertension and whose BP was adequately controlled during the measurement year	NQF 0018	
Cervical cancer screening	Percentage of women 21–64 years of age, who received one or more Pap tests to screen for cervical cancer	NQF 0032	
Chlamydia screening for women	Percentage of women 15–24 years of age who were identified as sexually active and who had at least one test for chlamydia during the measurement year	NQF 0033	
Use of appropriate medications for asthma	Percentage of patients 5–50 years of age who were identified as having persistent asthma and were appropriately prescribed medication during the measurement year. Report 3 age stratifications (5–11 years, 12–50 years, and total)	NQF 0036	
Low back pain: use of imaging studies	Percentage of patients with a primary diagnosis of low back pain who did not have an imaging study (plain x-ray, MRI, CT scan) within 28 days of diagnosis	NQF 0052	
Ischemic vascular disease (IVD): complete lipid panel and ldl control	Percentage of patients 18 years of age and older who were discharged alive for acute myocardial infarction (AMI), coronary artery bypass graft (CABG) or percutaneous transluminal coronary angioplasty (PTCA) from January 1–November 1 of the year before the measurement year, or who had a diagnosis of ischemic vascular disease (IVD) during the measurement year and the year before the measurement year and who had a complete lipid profile performed during the measurement year and whose LDL-C<100 mg/dL	NQF 0075	
Diabetes: hemoglobin A1c control (<8.0%)	Percentage of patients 18–75 years of age with diabetes (type 1 or type 2) who had hemoglobin A1c <8.0%	NQF 0575	

Abbreviations: ACC/AHA, American College of Cardiology/American Heart Association; CT, computed tomography; LVEF, left ventricular ejection fraction; MRI, magnetic resonance imaging; NQF, National Quality Forum; PQRI, Physician Quality Reporting Initiative.

year-after-year, by the end of 2016, you will have received up to $44,000 in incentive payments from Medicare FFS.

Scenario 3

You are a typical anesthesiologist in the United States who works wherever your anesthesia group assigns you each day. Today, for instance, you will be working in the operating room of a private hospital. Tomorrow, you will be based out of an ambulatory surgery center. As **Table 7** shows, only about 30% of the POS codes you submit to Medicare are 21 or 23. Consequently, you are not considered hospital-based because you do not meet the 90% threshold. As a non–hospital-based EP, you qualify for the CMS incentive payments for using the anesthesia information management systems (AIMS) at the hospitals, outpatient clinics, and ambulatory surgery centers where you work. Moreover, when you review the list of meaningful use criteria, you realize that you meet the exclusion criteria for several of them; the others, you believe you will be able to meet using certified EHR technology.

As illustrated in Scenario 3, the typical anesthesiologist in the United States will not be considered hospital-based and will therefore be eligible for the EHR incentive programs. In analyzing the Stage 1 meaningful use exclusion criteria (as shown in **Table 8**), anesthesiologist EPs should be granted exclusions for at least 2 of the core set criteria—(1) use computerized provider order entry for medication orders and (3) generate and transmit permissible prescriptions electronically—and at least 3 of those from the menu set: (1) implement drug-formulary checks, (10) capability to submit electronic data to immunization registries, and (12) capability to submit electronic syndromic surveillance data to public health agencies. As mentioned previously, each excluded criterion reduces the number of criteria that the EP must satisfy by one. Consequently, anesthesiologist EPs who meet the exclusion criteria for 3 menu set criteria need to choose only 2 more from the menu set to meet. In short, anesthesiologist EPs should be able to meet the remaining core set and 2 menu set criteria using certified AIMS EHR technology.

OPPORTUNITIES FOR ANESTHESIOLOGISTS

The HITECH Act's substantial positive and negative incentives are designed to encourage EPs, eligible hospitals, and CAHs to adopt and meaningfully use EHR

Table 7
Anesthesiologist Medicare Current Procedural Terminology (CPT) codes submitted in 2008

Place of Service (POS) Code	No. of CPT Codes Submitted	Percentage of Codes Submitted (%)
21: Inpatient Hospital	3,776,620	29.6
23: Emergency Room, Hospital	16,669	0.1
Total Hospital-Based	*3,793,289*	*29.7*
22: Outpatient Hospital	3,546,483	27.8
24: Ambulatory Surgery Center	1,954,336	15.3
11: Office	3,430,705	26.9
Other	27,972	0.2
Total Non–Hospital-Based	*8,959,496*	*70.3*
All codes	12,752,785	100.0

Data from the American Society of Anesthesiologists.

Table 8
Stage 1 meaningful use criteria effects on anesthesia EPs

Objective	Effect on Anesthesia EP
Core Set	
1. Use computerized provider order entry (CPOE) for medication orders directly entered by any licensed health care professional who can enter orders into the medical record per state, local, and professional guidelines	Exempt (write fewer than 100 prescriptions a year)
2. Implement drug-drug and drug-allergy interaction checks	Meet using AIMS (recognizing very few intraoperative drug-drug interactions exist)
3. Generate and transmit permissible prescriptions electronically (eRx)	Exempt (write fewer than 100 prescriptions a year)
4. Record the following demographics: (A) Preferred language, (B) Gender, (C) Race, (D) Ethnicity, (E) Date of birth	Meet using AIMS
5. Maintain an up-to-date problem list of current and active diagnoses	Meet using AIMS
6. Maintain active medication list	Meet using AIMS
7. Maintain active medication allergy list	Meet using AIMS
8. Record and chart changes in vital signs: (1) Height, (2) Weight, (3) Blood pressure, (4) Calculate and display the body mass index (BMI), (5) Plot and display growth charts for children 2 to 20 years old, including BMI	Meet using AIMS (recognizing that calculating/displaying growth charts is not part of the measure to meet this objective)
9. Record smoking status for patients 13 years old or older	Meet using AIMS
10. Implement 1 clinical decision support rule relevant to specialty or high clinical priority along with the ability to track compliance with that rule	Meet using AIMS
11. Report ambulatory clinical quality measures to CMS or, in the case of Medicaid EPs, the states	Meet using AIMS (recognizing that most of the measures are inapplicable)
12. Provide patients with an electronic copy of their health information (including diagnostic test results, problem list, medication lists, medication allergies) upon request	Meet using AIMS but potential for exemption if no requests for electronic copies of patient health information during the year
13. N/A for EPs	N/A
14. Provide clinical summaries for patients for each office visit	Exempt for the typical anesthesiologist (no office visits during the year)
15. Capability to exchange key clinical information (for example, problem list, medication list, medication allergies, diagnostic test results), among providers of care and patient-authorized entities electronically	Meet using AIMS
16. Protect electronic health information created or maintained by the certified EHR technology through the implementation of appropriate technical capabilities	Meet using AIMS

(continued on next page)

Table 8 (continued)	
Menu Set	
17. Implement drug-formulary checks	Exempt (write fewer than 100 prescriptions a year)
18. N/A for EPs	N/A
19. Incorporate clinical laboratory-test results into certified EHR technology as structured data	Meet using AIMS/hospital EHR
20. Generate lists of patients by specific conditions to use for quality improvement, reduction of disparities, research and outreach*	Meet using AIMS
21. Send reminders to patients per patient preference for preventive/follow-up care	Choose not to meet this one
22. Provide patients with timely electronic access to their health information (including lab results, problem list, medication lists, medication allergies) within 4 business days of the information being available to the EP	Meet using AIMS/hospital EHR
23. Use certified EHR technology to identify patient-specific education resources and provide those resources to the patient if appropriate	Choose not to meet this one
24. The EP, eligible hospital, or CAH who receives a patient from another setting of care or provider of care or believes an encounter is relevant should perform medication reconciliation	Meet using AIMS
25. The EP, eligible hospital, or CAH who transitions their patient to another setting of care or provider of care should provide summary of care record for each transition of care or referral	Meet using AIMS
26. Capability to submit electronic data to immunization registries or Immunization Information Systems and actual submission in accordance with applicable law and practice	Exempt (do not give immunizations)
27. N/A for EPs	N/A
28. Capability to submit electronic syndromic surveillance data to public health agencies and actual submission in accordance with applicable law and practice	Exempt (do not collect reportable syndromic information)

Abbreviations: AIMS, anesthesia information management systems; BMI, body mass index; CAH, critical access hospital; CMS, Centers for Medicare and Medicaid Services; EHR, electronic health record; EP, eligible professional; N/A, not applicable.

technology. In finalizing the meaningful use criteria, CMS was very responsive to feedback from the public regarding inapplicability of some of the criteria to certain medical specialties. In its final rule, CMS divided the criteria into 2 sets (including one with more flexibility and reduced requirements), provided exclusions, and eliminated those criteria that were considered unreasonable to require for Stage 1. The final rule from CMS is encouraging to the typical anesthesiologist who is not being considered as hospital-based and therefore eligible to receive incentive payments beginning in 2011.

As a field hailed for its high standards of quality and patient safety, and one that remains at the forefront of technological savvy, anesthesiology should embrace meaningful use. Besides adding some additional functionality to existing AIMS technology, none of the core meaningful use criteria are unreasonable requirements or significantly out of the typical anesthesiologist's scope of practice. Moreover, the standards, implementation specifications, and certification criteria for EHR technology help to standardize HIT in terms of vocabulary used, content exchange processes, privacy, and security, which promotes interoperability both between AIMS and a hospital's EHR and across different EHR systems. The implications of this improved information exchange are profound: improved patient safety and quality, enhanced communication among providers within and across fields, and increased opportunities for clinical outcomes and comparative effectiveness research. For anesthesiologists particularly, improved information exchange has the added bonus of simply making it easier to measure and convey all the work we already do.

Non–hospital-based anesthesiologists who do not currently use an AIMS have even more reason now to adopt and implement one. Anesthesiologists who adopt and meaningfully use certified EHR technology by 2015 can receive substantial monetary incentives of up to $44,000 from Medicare FFS or MA, or up to $63,750 from Medicaid. After 2015, the incentive for anesthesiologists is to avoid the indefinite downward payment adjustments for not being meaningful EHR users. These positive and negative monetary incentives by CMS are a solid solution to the continual barrier to EHR and AIMS implementation of a lack of clear return-on-investment.[1] These incentives are in addition to the other evidence-based factors that result in a positive return-on-investment from the adoption of AIMS: reducing anesthetic-related drug costs, improving staff scheduling and reducing staffing costs, increasing anesthesia billing and capture of anesthesia-related charges, and increasing hospital reimbursement through improved hospital coding.[2,3]

Moreover, anesthesiologists may be able to benefit from supporting hospitals in their adoption and meaningful use of certified EHR technology. Under Medicare FFS and MA, eligible hospitals (ie, those located in the 50 states and the District of Columbia) that adopt and meaningfully use EHR by 2015 can receive up to 4 years of incentive payments according to the formula in **Fig. 1**: *Medicare incentive payment = initial amount × Medicare share × transition factor*. After 2015, eligible hospitals that are not meaningful EHR users are subject to penalties of one-quarter, one-half, and three-quarter reductions to their market basket update for inpatient hospital services in 2015, 2016, and 2017 and beyond, respectively. Eligible hospitals that fail to report data on quality measures are subject to another one-quarter reduction. Owing to the diminishing transition factor in the formula, eligible hospitals must become meaningful users of EHR by 2013 to take full advantage of the CMS incentive programs. If anesthesiologists can use AIMS to help their hospitals meet their meaningful use requirements, especially sooner than later, then the hospitals are much more likely to support the purchase of AIMS, thus eliminating a significant cost that anesthesiologists would have had to bear themselves.

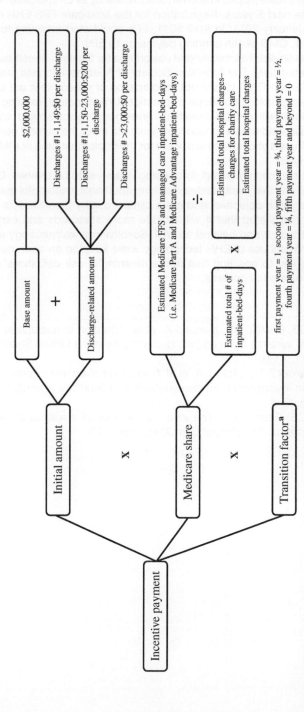

Fig. 1. Medicare incentive payment calculation for eligible hospitals. [a] If the eligible hospital's first payment year is 2014, the applicable transition factor is ¾ for the first payment year, ½ for the second payment year, and ¼ for the third payment year. If the first payment year is 2015, the applicable transition factor is ½ for the first payment year and ¼ for the second payment year.

Regardless of how individual anesthesiologists feel about adopting EHR, the reality is that the government has stepped in and required its use by all EPs, eligible hospitals, and CAHs within the next 5 years. Registration for the Medicare FFS EHR incentive program began in January 2011. In April 2011, EPs could start attesting to the use of EHR. In May 2011, CMS began sending payments to EPs.

Now that CMS has finalized its meaningful use criteria for Stage 1, anesthesiologists should proceed strategically. The American Society of Anesthesiologists has already reached out to CMS and ONC to attempt modification of criteria that are out of an operating room anesthesiologist's scope of practice. Unfortunately, existing Stage 1 criteria or exemptions will not be modified. Anesthesiologists should work with AIMS vendors to ensure adequate functionality exists to meet the current certification criteria. Anesthesiologists should also advocate for the implementation of AIMS by the facilities they work with.

Although Stage 1 has been finalized, future stages are yet to be defined. CMS has mentioned in its final rule that it anticipates requiring additional meaningful use criteria, harder measures for each objective, and more clinical quality measures for Stage 2 and beyond. ONC has stated that it will include more standards and certification criteria for EHR in Stage 2 and beyond as well. Solidifying anesthesiology as a field that supports meaningful use of EHR technology while keeping an open dialog with CMS and ONC are key to ensuring that future meaningful use definitions continue to consider its interests and concerns.

REFERENCES

1. Egger Halbeis CB, Epstein RH, Macario A, et al. Adoption of anesthesia information management systems by academic departments in the United States. Anesth Analg 2008;107:1323–9.
2. O'Sullivan CT, Dexter F, Lubarsky DA, et al. Evidence-based management assessment of return on investment from anesthesia information management systems. AANA J 2007;75:43–8.
3. Egger Halbeis CB, Epstein RH. The value proposition of anesthesia information management systems. Anesthesiol Clin 2008;26:665–79.

Quality Improvement Using Automated Data Sources: The Anesthesia Quality Institute

Richard P. Dutton, MD, MBA[a],*, Andrew DuKatz, MS[b]

KEYWORDS

- Quality management
- Anesthesiology information management system
- AIMS • Registry • Outcomes

QUALITY IMPROVEMENT IN ANESTHESIOLOGY

Improving the quality of health care, including anesthesia, is a fundamentally simple cycle of observing outcomes, analyzing causation, making changes in care, and reobserving. The first step, observation, assumes the collection of data. The second step, analysis, defines the data that will be needed, which falls broadly into 3 categories, as shown in **Fig. 1**, and can be described as what we start with, what we do, and what happens. Risk factors are those elements of a case that are in place at the start, and are largely beyond the anesthesiologist's control. Risk factors include data such as patient age and sex, preexisting diseases and physiology, the kind of operation to be performed, and even systemic variables such as the presence or absence of surgical residents. Process data includes all that the anesthesiologist brings to the equation: the type of anesthesia performed, the specific medications used, the quantity of fluid or blood products administered, the monitors applied, and the maintenance targets for blood pressure, heart rate, glucose, hematocrit, and other measures of physiology. Outcomes are the real data of interest to patients and regulators, and these reflect the interaction between risk and process. Outcomes can be patient centered (eg, mortality, postoperative nausea and vomiting) or system centered (eg, cost of care, length of stay). Outcomes can be durable changes in function (eg,

The authors have no conflicts of interest to disclose.
[a] Anesthesia Quality Institute, 520 North NW Highway, Park Ridge, IL 60068, USA
[b] MS-3, University of Maryland School of Medicine, 22 South Greene Street, Baltimore, MD 21201, USA
* Corresponding author.
E-mail address: r.dutton@asahq.org

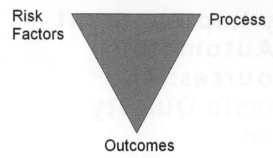

Fig. 1. The quality triangle, illustrating the data required to improve anesthesia care.

a myocardial infarct) or surrogates associated with such a change (eg, postoperative increase of troponin level). Comparing risk-adjusted outcomes associated with different process decisions is at the heart of both scientific research and anesthesia quality management (QM).

In the information age, the passive acquisition and processing of electronic data offers new opportunities for quality improvement that were not present even a decade ago. As discussed in the article by Kheterpal and Tremper elsewhere in this issue, it is now possible to envision a future state of anesthesia practice that is completely paper-less, from preoperative assessment through intraoperative record to postoperative collection of outcomes. Transition from paper to digital records creates the possibility for automated accumulation of anesthesia case data at an unprecedented scope and scale. The Multicenter Perioperative Outcomes Group (MPOG; discussed in the article by Sachin Kheterpal elsewhere in this issue) is one effort to leverage this capacity for academic purposes. The National Anesthesia Clinical Outcomes Registry (NACOR) of the Anesthesia Quality Institute (AQI) is another.

THE NEED FOR ANESTHESIA OUTCOMES DATA

Coincident with the increased capacities of digital record keeping, there has been a steady increase in regulatory pressure to document the quality and value of health care. The Federal Government, which directly or indirectly funds more than half of the health care provided in the United States, has implemented a series of laws and regulations designed to encourage the quality and financial efficiency of health care. One example is the Physician Quality Reporting System (PQRS), which offers partici-pating physicians a small incentive bonus to payments from Medicare if they can document compliance with specialty-specific, evidence-based processes of care that are known to be associated with improved patient outcomes. Three of these stan-dards currently apply to anesthesiologists, all related to prevention of surgical site infections: administration of preoperative prophylactic antibiotics in a timely fashion, use of a best-practice bundle of techniques for central line placement, and mainte-nance of patient normothermia during and after major surgeries.[1] Another example is the recently announced physician incentive for meaningful use of health care infor-mation technology. Although in its infancy, this program will provide financial incen-tives to doctors, possibly including anesthesiologists, who have committed to the use of electronic record-keeping systems (discussed elsewhere in this issue). The Center for Medicare and Medicaid Services (CMS) has initiated a program whereby physicians can meet their requirements for PQRS standards by contributing their data to qualifying electronic case registries, and has made contribution through this mechanism easier than independent (claims-based) documentation.[2]

Noteworthy in the government roll-out of both PQRS and meaningful use is the concept that the incentives of today will transform, in the next 5 to 10 years, into penalties for those physicians who are not participating. Other regulatory pressures are coming to bear on anesthesiologists as well. The Joint Commission, the deemed certifying body of most US hospitals, has made the Focused Professional Practice Evaluation (FPPE) and the Ongoing Professional Practice Evaluation (OPPE) requirements for all physicians working in a surveyed hospital. FPPE is required for each new physician coming on staff, as well as for credentialing existing providers to perform new procedures. It asks the hospital the simple question, "How do you know this physician is qualified?" Previously, this might have been answered through reference to documented completion of a residency and perhaps certification by a specialty board, but now the expectation is that it will include direct observation of patient care and analysis of outcomes. OPPE asks the equivalent question for existing staff members: "How do you know this doctor is still capable?" OPPE similarly expects ongoing documentation of outcomes from current practice. Both of these programs merely reflect the emerging standards for maintenance of certification that all professional boards have now adopted. Maintenance of Certification in Anesthesiology (MOCA) is required for any anesthesiologist to be board certified in 2000 or later, and is voluntary (but strongly encouraged by state and local hospital requirements) for others. What began as a simple written recertification test has now become a multiyear process that involves documentation of ongoing continuing medical education and completion of a personal practice assessment that closely mirrors the FPPE and OPPE process.

These emerging regulatory requirements will have a profound effect on the practice of anesthesiology in the United States. Recognizing both the need to assist its members and the enormous potential of digital case information to improve patient care, the American Society of Anesthesiologists (ASA) chartered the AQI in 2009 to provide a new resource for anesthesia practice benchmarking nationwide.

DATA AVAILABLE

In creating NACOR, the AQI focused on the potential for collection of existing digital data. Operations began with a review of what was already available. Although there are literally billions of pages on the Internet, most information is not organized in a way that makes it tailored for data analysis. The usefulness of online databases is generally based on the format of their stored data, which includes unstructured, structured, and semistructured information. Clinically oriented databases such as those that contain drug information are often unstructured.[3] These databases are human readable but require a human to translate the information if analysis is required. Structured data, which limits the data stored in a field to a specific list (eg, a predefined values) or format (eg, whole numbers), simplifies automated analysis, filtering, and sorting. For instance, the Entrez Gene database (http://www.ncbi.nlm.nih.gov/gene) provides specific information related to the name, lineage, and location for genes. Another example, although not tailored to medicine, is online travel databases, which would not be useful if the user could not search for a flight based on date, city pair, or airline. In addition, a semistructured database like PubMed (http://www.ncbi.nlm.nih.gov/pubmed/) includes discrete values for items like the publication name, date, and page numbers, but unstructured information in the form of the abstract. A list of common medical databases can be found at http://www.nlm.nih.gov/databases/.

Unstructured data may be easier for clinicians to use, but is harder to manipulate in the digital world. Structured data are easy to transmit, report, and analyze, but may lose precision when translated from original, unstructured data entries. Clinical information of interest to anesthesiologists comes in both structured form (eg, vital signs) and unstructured form (eg, procedure notes or comments on the anesthetic record). There are 4 major sources for digital data of relevance to anesthesiology:

- Anesthesia professional billing systems. These systems are in use in virtually every anesthesia practice (or the professional management company that supports them) and are highly structured, but limited in content. In the simplest form, the billing system includes only a provider, a procedure (usually by Current Procedural Terminology [CPT] code), and a duration.
- Anesthesia information management systems (AIMS). These electronic medical records for the OR include structured capture of most intraoperative process data: vital signs, medications, times, and fluids. AIMS also include unstructured or semistructured reporting of events (eg, induction, intubation, emergence). The relative degrees of structured, semistructured, and unstructured data in AIMS is based on the vendor, configuration of the software, and the practice patterns of the providers using the system. AIMS are in use in 10% to 20% of (mostly larger and academic) US hospitals; many more facilities are in the process of buying or installing an AIMS.
- Hospital electronic records. There are useful data on patient demographics and on short-term outcomes available in digital hospital records, including laboratory values before and after surgery, diagnostic codes before and after surgery, medications used, and length-of-stay information. Availability and constructive interconnection of these systems is highly variable across facilities. In some hospitals, the AIMS is purchased from the same vendor as the hospital's electronic health care records (EHR) system. In these environments, the AIMS is completely integrated into hospital EHR and both draws from and contributes to the overall patient record. Other hospitals use custom-developed interfaces to share data between AIMS and the EHR. In this scenario, the AIMS and EHR software are sold by different vendors, thus preventing seamless integration between the systems. In other settings, AIMS may be isolated from other systems and contributes little more than a printout at the end of the case.
- Anesthesia QM systems. These systems are home-grown programs, databases (often using Microsoft Access), or simple spreadsheets created to capture outcome information collected by the hospital, anesthesia group, or a specific anesthetic service (eg, pediatrics). They are typically populated by providers at the end of a case, or by Postanesthetic Care Unit (PACU) or clinic nurses trained to call back patients 24 to 48 hours after surgery and screen them for outcomes of interest. Variability in timing, topics, and definitions is high. A few practices are beginning to offer their software for sale to others, but there is no single system in common use.

REGISTRY MODELS

Up to the present day, most successful registries of clinical data have been based on a similar development model: identifying a population to focus on, listing the variables of interest, recruiting groups to contribute data, and manual abstraction of information from patient medical records into the registry. Examples of this model of registry that may be familiar to anesthesiologists include the National Surgical Quality Improvement Project (NSQIP), the National Trauma Data Bank, the Society of Thoracic Surgeons Database, and the Malignant Hypothermia Association of the United States registry (MHAUS). Modern technology can make it easier to identify patients, and can facilitate the work of the data abstractors in entering data. The data entered can be precisely defined, and the abstractors (usually nurses employed by the hospital's QM office) can be trained in a uniform fashion. These advantages are balanced by the time and cost of data acquisition, which can be substantial. Because every data element must move through the human filter of the abstractor, there are limits on the number of patients that can be included and the number of data points that can be captured. Participation in these registries is expensive ($150,000 per year on average for NSQIP hospitals) and the sample is therefore biased toward larger and more academic hospitals.

In building NACOR, the AQI sought to develop a different model, based on periodic transfer of case-specific data directly from one electronic system to another. This model takes advantage of the ongoing implementation (and interconnection) of health care information technology in anesthesia practice, and, in theory, should be far more cost-effective than a registry dependent on individual human case abstraction. Other potential advantages of this model include:

- All cases are reported, instead of a potentially biased subset
- Many more data points per case can be reported and archived
- Data flow is automatic and passive
- Uniform definitions can be applied in the electronic transfer process
- Data from different systems can be linked
- Automated cleaning and audit functions can be built in
- Technology solutions developed for one institution can be easily ported to other clients of the same vendor. Automated reports and trending over time can be built into the system
- New data elements and revised definitions can be easily added, and data collection can be made deeper over time as facility and practice capabilities expand.

The use of AIMS to store and transmit data to NACOR is particularly advantageous in anesthesia. First, the 80/20 rule applies to anesthesia data collection: 80% of the data captured by anesthetic providers are already standardized (even if the formatting or meaning is slightly different), making it simple to share common data elements. Second, market consolidation among AIMS vendors has led to only a handful of major vendors. The use of standard AIMS software eases the incorporation of AIMS data into NACOR, because the mapping of data elements from the vendor software to NACOR needs to occur only once. Third, the analysis of large data sets can be used to influence and justify future data collection needs.

Compared with the traditional model, a new model registry will offer several challenges as well. These challenges must be identified as early in the process as possible, so that steps can be taken to mitigate their impact. First, the capacity to roll up electronic data at the national level requires the existence of that data in the first place. Some data (eg, administrative billing information) are already universally available. Some data (eg, anesthesia process information from AIMS) are available in some practices but not others, although all groups are moving toward increasing use of electronic records. In addition, there are some data (typically postoperative patient outcomes) that are rarely collected in the first place and, when collected, may not be recorded in an accessible electronic system. Overcoming this problem will require collective effort across the profession. Motivation will arise not only from an increasing desire to understand the best way to care for patients but also from increasing regulatory requirements to measure and report on patient-centered outcomes.

Second, the practice patterns of individual anesthesiology providers (whether anesthesiologists, residents, or Certified Registered Nurse Anesthesiologists) may possibly affect the quality and quantity of data collected. Although AIMS automatically captures physiologic and ventilation data and uses electronic forms to collect other perioperative data, the anesthesiologists' professional experience and their exposure to AIMS may have an impact on the collected data. For instance, a provider who rotates among hospitals may only use AIMS once a month and never gain complete comfort using the system. This approach contrasts with the precision and uniformity of a nurse data abstractor.

Third, the choice of a specific AIMS vendor and the corresponding configuration of the AIMS may affect the mapping of data to NACOR. For instance, certain anesthesiology groups may be interested in capturing anatomic details related to the intubation process, whereas others may require far fewer data. Even within anesthesiology groups, the level of data captured may vary based on the practice patterns of the provider. The variability in the types of data collected could potentially affect the ability to perform data analysis systematically.

Fourth, most anesthesia-relevant electronic data exist at the present in various proprietary formats. In order for NACOR to accept these data, they must first be normalized into a standard schema or format. As shown in **Fig. 2**, translation of data (sometimes called mapping) can occur at either end of the communications pipeline, but requires a significant commitment of knowledgeable technical resources to accomplish. Translation further requires that the meaning of each data element be clearly and unambiguously defined. For instance, data accumulation would be compromised if 2 different organizations did not have the same understanding of the ASA Physical Status system or used different terms to specify this variable (such as Arabic vs Roman numerals). Another simple example that highlights the ambiguity of collecting even simple data elements is the specification of the units for height (inches or centimeters) or weight (pounds or kilograms) that are required to calculate body mass index (BMI). Even in a single hospital system, different services may not communicate this information consistently. If the EHR does not include the units while transmitting the relevant data, there is no way to calculate the BMI. Thus, a common vocabulary is required to successfully fill the registry.

The National Center for Clinical Outcomes Research (NCCOR) recognized these challenges in the course of developing their registry in the 1990s. As a result of this

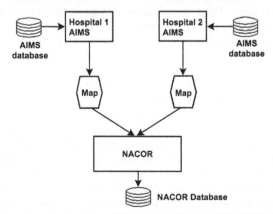

Fig. 2. Mapping data from various providers to the National Center for Clinical Outcomes Research (NCCOR). Each hospital has installed an AIMS from a different vendor. In order for NACOR to store the data, there is a mapping utility that converts the data to a common format.

project, the Anesthesia Patient Safety Foundation committed to establishing a common data format for anesthetic providers. The original Data Dictionary Task Force (DDTF) (established in 2000) merged several times with international organizations and now exists as a subproject within SNOMED (Standard NOmenclature for MEDicine), a comprehensive standard for medical terminology developed and used by the Federal Government. In turn, SNOMED partnered with the International Health Terminology Standards Development Organization (IHTSDO) to create a worldwide common language for medicine, and the DDTF has transitioned into the International Organization for Terminology in Anesthesia (IOTA). The development of this anesthetic ontology (in simplistic terms, an electronic representation of the perioperative and anesthetic record) has required a cooperative effort between practitioners and established AIMS vendors.[4–6] Future versions of AIMS software will hopefully incorporate these standards.

Where possible, the AQI has embraced existing standard definitions, such as those developed by IOTA, as the basis for its schema. Where a standard definition for a desired variable does not exist in IOTA, the AQI has either found a common definition developed by a national consensus organization (eg, the procedural times glossary of the American Association of Clinical Directors)[7] or developed its own, based on the best information available. The AQI has deliberately chosen to make its definitions, and the entire schema, publicly and prominently available on its Web site.[8,9] This has been of use to EHR vendors, and will hopefully encourage the universal adoption of common definitions.

Even when commercial EHR vendors use different definitions, mapping of most data is still possible. The MPOG has successfully created a research database with inputs from multiple different AIMS (see the article elsewhere in this issue). Walsh and colleagues[10] at the Massachusetts General Hospital have used Extensible Markup Language (XML) to link anesthetic data from their AIMS into the National Surgical Quality Improvement Program, successfully combining anesthesia process information with perioperative patient risk data and postoperative surgical outcomes.

BENEFITS OF ELECTRONIC ANESTHESIA DATA

Understanding the potential of the AQI to improve the practice of anesthesiology depends on first understanding the benefits of electronic data collection at the local hospital level. Although commercially available anesthesiology information management systems (AIMS) have existed for more than 20 years, the rate of adoption in anesthesiology practices has been low because it has taken time and technical evolution for them to realize their potential. However, the process of adoption does seem to be accelerating, and will likely do so even faster in the next decade in response to government pressure on providers and facilities to adopt EHR. A survey within the last 3 years estimated that 5% to 10% of US hospitals have adopted AIMS,[11] whereas 44% of US academic medical centers have implemented AIMS or committed to do so.[12]

Early AIMS were developed for their ability to reduce the workload of the anesthesia provider by capturing physiologic data automatically and printing it on paper.[13] However, as technology has evolved, the benefits of an AIMS now include revenue generation (automated support of billing functions), quality assurance, satisfaction of regulatory mandates, decision and research support, and enhancing the ability of the provider to focus on the patient.[14–19] Despite these perceived benefits of an AIMS, possible reasons for the low rate of adoption have been an inability to justify the return on investment (ROI), the inherent complexity of the system, challenges related to system integration, inability to acquire funding, and substantial ongoing operating and maintenance costs.[20,21] For instance, the computation of ROI for the purchase and installation of an AIMS is often dependent on unrealistic and difficult-to-quantify assumptions.[20] Furthermore, the standard AIMS configuration may not meet an organization's needs, resulting in costly development of custom capabilities.[19]

One challenge for AIMS adopters, similar to adopters of any other information technology product, is learning to view AIMS as a tool and not as a complete solution.[18] Although tailored to the anesthesia environment, the benefits of AIMS have taken time to accrue, as early adopters have increasingly used core AIMS features such as perioperative data collection and workflow management (eg, templates and event alarms).

Because of the quality and quantity of data captured within AIMS, retrospective data analysis has been used for adverse event planning,[22] identifying patient risk factors,[23] economic benefits,[24] and risk management.[25] A deficiency in voluntary adverse event reporting has been shown by scanning AIMS records to automatically detect adverse events,[22] and an association has been found between the existence of these adverse events and the occurrence of inpatient mortality.[26] AIMS data have been used to statistically calculate perioperative and intraoperative risk factors, including hypotension in women undergoing cesarean section using spinal anesthesia,[23] the prediction of antiemetic rescue treatment as an indicator for postoperative nausea and vomiting,[27] and a model to predict intraoperative cardiovascular events.[28] The potential to use AIMS data in epidemiologic studies has been shown in a study that showed undertreatment and gender differences in the medical treatment of patients with coronary artery disease who presented for surgical treatment.[29] A bayesian model concluded that a 20% to 25% reduction in average time from case end to extubation can be realized when using desflurane compared with sevoflurane.[24] In addition, atypical drug transactions recorded in AIMS have been used to discover drug diversion by providers.[25]

Retrospective data analysis has the potential to influence professional liability.[30] Through a statistical analysis of the minimum heart rate, maximum heart rate, minimum arterial oxyhemoglobin saturation (SaO_2), minimum mean arterial pressure (MAP), maximum MAP, decrease in MAP, and increase in MAP, the investigators of one study calculated reference limits for vital signs during cesarean section. Based on their data, the investigators suggested that adverse outcomes were unlikely to be caused by the anesthesiologist as long as the vital signs remained within these calculated reference limits. This theory has yet to be tested in a prospective trial, but offers an interesting look at the profession's future ability to define normal and effective practice.

In addition to retrospective data analysis, the prospective capture of physiologic data has been leveraged in novel ways for operating room management,[31] compliance,[32] risk management,[33] and revenue generation. The accuracy of operating room occupancy can be inferred in real time from vital sign data transmitted by AIMS.[31] In this study, a bayesian method was used to estimate the remaining case time by incorporating historical case duration data, scheduled case duration and elapsed times, and a series of pop-up messages displayed on the AIMS screen.[34] In another study, an algorithm was developed to trigger an electronic alarm within the AIMS when pulsatile flow returned after disabling monitor alarms during cardiopulmonary bypass.[33]

Automated intraoperative monitoring of physiologic data has been used to improve compliance and revenue generation.[32] In this study, an algorithm was developed that monitored the AIMS record and determined whether the anesthesia provider was using an invasive arterial blood pressure catheter. An e-mail and page was sent to providers who had not added a procedure note during or after surgery. The control group and study group had compliance rates of 84% and 99% respectively, showing the potential to identify increased revenue opportunities from previously unbilled procedures. Similarly, nonphysiologic perioperative data have been scanned intraoperatively using AIMS. In one study, text messages were automatically sent to providers who had not completed the allergy field in the AIMS record, improving the compliance rate for completion of this specific field.[35]

Multiple studies have shown the potential of AIMS to enhance anesthesia workflow for perioperative and quality assurance data collection,[36] staff recall,[37] and revenue generation.[38] Handheld computers have been successfully integrated into the data collection process before surgery and during pain rounds.[36,39,40] Using a list of predefined indicators on an electronic form, the collection rate of quality assurance data increased from 48% to 78%.[36] AIMS have been used to convert a manual phone tree for mass casualty recall to an automated system by automatically sending SMS messages to providers' cell phones.[37] In addition, a decrease in billing time from 3.0 days to 1.1 days was shown in a study that used an algorithm to continuously poll the AIMS database for documentation errors and then alert providers via page.[38]

A common workflow feature of an AIMS is the ability to trigger perioperative and intraoperative event reminders. This capability has been used to decrease the incidence of deviations from standard of care, such as reminding clinicians to administer prophylactic antibiotics to prevent surgical site infection (SSI).[41,42] The use of a multiprong strategy for disseminating prophylactic antibiotic compliance results to providers improved compliance from 69% to 92% in one study.[41] First, e-mail was used to provide individual provider feedback. Second, departmental results were posted in highly visible locations. Third, department leaders sought out staff who had repeated lapses. Based on an analysis of the data, anesthesia providers were instructed to modify the timing of prophylactic antibiotic administration to increase compliance (eg, dosing shortly after entering the room rather than during surgical prep).

Similar to other information technology implementations, challenges occur during the adoption of an AIMS. The quality of captured data is affected by the configuration of the system. The use of free text fields instead of structured text fields and a lack of question linking (eg, use of follow-on questions based on answers to previous questions) has resulted in decreased compliance and usefulness of data.[43] The automatic reconciliation of dispensed versus administered medications may be impractical because of data entry issues with AIMS and challenges integrating interfaces with the pharmacy system.[44] The ergonomics of an additional monitor and keyboard in the operating room is critical for user acceptance. At one hospital, a rear-view mirror was used to maintain visual contact with the patient in a tightly spaced endoscopic suite.[45] There have been several preventable malpractice claims in which the fault lay with either technical glitches or changes in anesthesia workflow. In one claim, staff did not recognize the loss of incoming AIMS data and did not manually enter captured data from the physiologic monitors.[46] Another claim described how the AIMS audit trail was used to suggest that an attending physician was not present at extubation because of preattested documentation.[47] Overall, however, AIMS are believed to reduce the risk of litigation by offering more complete documentation, increased legibility, and fewer lost records.

BENEFITS OF NACOR

The purpose of a national registry of anesthesia case information is to multiply the local benefits of an AIMS (described earlier) across hundreds of anesthesia practices and health care facilities and the millions of anesthetics performed in the United States each year. Data from NACOR will be used for quality improvement, comparative effectiveness research, and national advocacy.

The most immediate use of AQI data will be on behalf of the anesthesia practices participating in NACOR data collection. A survey conducted by Audet and colleagues[7] found that only 33% of providers receive feedback in the form of data on the quality of the care they deliver to patients. By participating with NACOR, these groups will receive regular reports from the AQI that summarize their own case data in a standardized format and then benchmark aspects of their practice to an anonymous cohort of peer groups. This process will be done either for the practice as a whole or for individual facilities that the group covers. For example anesthesia time for an upper abdominal laparoscopy case might be compared within cohorts of ambulatory surgery centers, private inpatient hospitals, and academic medical centers. The mean and standard deviation of each center's cases would be displayed on a chart that ranks the centers from shortest to longest time. High outliers would be those centers with case times significantly shorter than the norm, whereas low outliers would be the opposite. Low outliers will benefit from knowledge of their standing, thus motivating efforts to improve, which could include internal efforts to improve anesthesia processes and practice, possibly drawing on resources provided by the ASA and AQI (eg, guidelines for preoperative testing), as well as use of the data to make external changes (eg, using the data as a lever to persuade the hospital to hire more housekeepers).

In time, AQI data will become a rich source for retrospective clinical research in anesthesiology, especially when comparing outcomes in similar groups of patients treated in 2 different ways (eg, regional vs general anesthesia for total hip arthroplasty). This comparative effectiveness research differs from the more traditional (and more precise) prospective randomized clinical trial because it is not possible to control for all of the biases that may influence any given clinical decision (eg, if sicker patients were more likely to receive regional anesthesia). Some of these biases can be identified and managed in the data collected (eg, by adjusting results based on ASA physical status) and some cannot. However, comparative effectiveness research enables the study of much larger numbers of patients than prospective trials and has an advantage in applicability because it is based in real-world practice. The US government is increasingly interested in the results of comparative effectiveness research to guide decisions about which procedures, processes, and medications to reimburse. The ability of the AQI to support academic uses of its data depends in large part on the depth and density of what is collected. As links to hospital EHR become more robust, it will become progressively easier to collect important risk-adjustment information such as comorbid conditions, preoperative laboratory values, and past medical history.

Data from NACOR will become an important resource for the leaders of ASA and for its committees, subspecialty societies, and foundations (**Fig. 3**). Aggregated national data will provide an understanding of the kinds and quantity of anesthetics performed, the most common cases done and populations served, and the overall safety of anesthesia practice. Identification of significant variations in outcome will prompt development of practice advisories and guidelines. Knowledge of which complications are most common, in which populations of patients, will guide both safety efforts and clinical research. NACOR will facilitate the ongoing work of other groups and individuals interested in anesthesia outcomes by providing, for example, denominator information to go with the malpractice numerators collected by the Closed Claims project. There is also the prospect of linking data from NACOR to the database and registry projects of

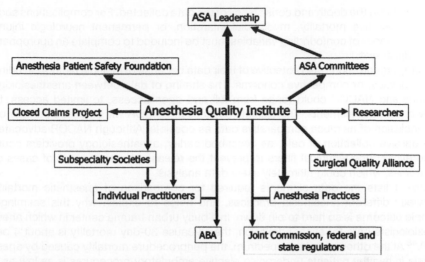

Fig. 3. AQI reporting of data from the NACOR.

other specialties, which will be done in the short term by synchronizing data definitions and electronic formats, and in the long term by actual exchange of matched (but still not identified) data.

POTENTIAL PITFALLS IN THE AQI PROCESS

Although the goals and approach of the AQI would seem a natural fit for the information age, there are some potential pitfalls that have to be overcome. For example, encouraging the collection of postoperative outcome information will increase the apparent rate of complications by including events that had not previously been discovered or reported. This effect can hamper the movement of professional culture toward one of open and honest reporting, particularly if short-term results are used publicly by opponents of the process. A similar impediment can arise from publicity surrounding isolated bad outcomes. Although management by anecdote is never a good strategy for QM systems, there exists a strong potential in human nature for hysterical response to negative events, which can include a desire to blame the bearer of bad news (in this case the AQI).

Another pitfall can arise from overeager analysis of collected data. By their nature, anesthesiologists are used to seeing rapid results from their actions. Although successful medical registries of the past have taken as long as 7 years to achieve useful results, it is likely that the AQI will be expected to begin reporting far sooner than this. Judgment and restraint will be required to avoid releasing data that are not well understood. For serious complications (fortunately rare in anesthesiology) this will require large numbers of cases, documented at sufficient depth of reporting and consistency of definition, to adequately interpret the results. Because anesthesia is a service industry, our outcomes are closely linked to factors brought to the table by our patients, our surgeons and our systems. Even an outcome as innocuous as postoperative nausea and vomiting is strongly confounded by the nature of the practice, and will be higher in a group with more strabismus and endometrial surgery than in one dealing mostly with older orthopedic patients. Reporting intelligently on such an outcome requires adjustment for preoperative risk; risk adjustment in turn requires an increase in the depth and consistency of the data collected. For complications such as perioperative mortality, myocardial infarction, or permanent neurologic injury, a huge number of confounding variables must be included to complete an appropriate risk adjustment.

Many organizations are protective of their data because of multiple factors including legal, privacy, or competitive concerns. The sharing of data between anesthesiology groups and NACOR could range from full and open access, to limited access, to only a few data elements. The ultimate success of NACOR will be based partially on the inclusion of as much comparative data as possible. Although NACOR advocates the passive collection of data, as described earlier, anesthesiology providers could theoretically use technical filters to prevent the release of certain types of cases or outcomes, which could ultimately skew data analysis.

Box 1 lists the data elements required for comparison of anesthetic mortality between different anesthesia practices, and helps to explain why this seemingly simple outcome is so hard to pin down. In a busy urban trauma center in which anesthesiologists care for every admission, the all-cause 30-day mortality is about 4 per 100.[48] At the other end of the spectrum, the periprocedure mortality caused by anesthesia in healthy patients undergoing elective ambulatory procedures is as low as 7 per million,[49] or 4 orders of magnitude different. Ironically, the trauma publication shows that the center's risk-adjusted mortality is among the best ever reported, and

---

Box 1
Calculating mortality for anesthesia

Although an obvious choice, calculation of mortality that allows comparison between practices is hard to do well, and illustrates several of the pitfalls inherent in the use of registry data.

1. Definitions must be consistent between practices

    a. Time to death: intraoperative, perioperative, less than 24 hours, less than 48 hours, less than 30 days?

    b. Patients included: every case? Every nonemergent case? Organ donors?

    c. Relationship to anesthesia: all cause? Anesthesia-related only? Who decides?

2. All cases must be included. Because the event (death) is rare, any missing event has an exaggerated effect on the final analysis

    a. No exclusion of some cases (automated passive systems help avoid this bias)

    b. Unknown mortality status must be investigated, not simply dropped. Missing data can be significant

3. Risk adjustment is required, to account for as many potential confounders as possible. Useful data include:

    a. Patient age and sex

    b. ASA physical status

    c. Scheduled surgery

    d. Emergency versus elective cases

    e. Comorbid conditions

    f. Preoperative medication use

    g. Preoperative laboratory values

    h. Preoperative physiology (vital signs or other diagnostics)

has improved significantly in the past decade, whereas the ambulatory publication expressed concern about an excess mortality for procedures performed in physician's offices. For outcomes that are more subjectively determined than mortality (eg, postoperative pain), the difficulty in creating meaningful comparisons becomes even greater, and the quantity and quality of data required to do it well becomes even larger.

The final pitfall inherent in any electronic system is the principle of garbage in, garbage out. Although the AQI can and will encourage practices to collect outcome data and report it using standard methods and standard definitions, the quality of NACOR ultimately depends on the quality of data collected at the patient level. If there is no recontact with the patient following PACU discharge, then no data can exist. If queries are imprecise or superficial, then data will be fuzzy. If outright fraud occurs, perhaps the result of overzealous pursuit of government incentives or a desire to gain a commercial advantage, then the validity of the system as a whole is threatened. There will always be a need for human review of submissions, and for a random auditing mechanism. The continuous and automated nature of NACOR offers some advantages in identifying suspect data through screening for statistically improbable results. In turn, this screening will allow for targeted auditing by human eyes, which will be necessary as NACOR matures. The deterrent value of these mechanisms should be sufficient to preserve the overall quality of AQI data, as well as a willingness to publicly confront those who are cheating the system, but eternal vigilance will be required.

SUMMARY

The AQI has created the NACOR based on the premise that anesthesia practice, and health care in general, will become increasingly digitized in the next 2 decades. NACOR will be the next-level destination for automatically generated data from AIMS and related EHR, and will enable data analysis and benchmarking based on millions of cases nationally rather than thousands of cases locally. Data from NACOR will provide the leaders of anesthesiology with aggregated information about national practice, and will enable more precise estimation of the scope of care provided by anesthesiologists, the overall effectiveness of that care, and the rate of serious complications. The AQI itself has the potential to become the central source in anesthesiology for defining process and outcome. Perhaps even more importantly, the AQI will be able to leverage data from NACOR to create change at the local level, by exporting best practices from high-performing practices to those with deficiencies. Less flashy than avoiding rare extreme outcomes, routine improvement in outcomes such as emergence time, hospital length of stay, postoperative nausea and vomiting, and severe pain will help to cement the reputation of anesthesiology as a safe and patient-oriented profession.

REFERENCES

1. US Department of Health and Human Services. 2010 PQRI Measures List. Baltimore (MD): Centers for Medicare and Medicaid Services; 2009.
2. Tavener M, US Department of Health and Human Services. Medicare and Medicaid programs; electronic health record incentive program. Baltimore (MD): Centers for Medicare and Medicaid Services; 2010.
3. Available at: http://www.nlm.nih.gov/medlineplus/druginformation.html. Accessed June 14, 2011.
4. Monk T. Available at: http://www.apsf.org/initiatives/infosys.mspx. Accessed June 4, 2010.

5. Available at: http://www.nlm.nih.gov/research/umls/Snomed/snomed_main.html. Accessed June 4, 2010.
6. Available at: http://www.apsf.org/initiatives/data_dictionary.mspx. Accessed June 4, 2010.
7. Audet AM, Doty MM, Shamasdin J, et al. Measure, learn, and improve: physicians' involvement in quality improvement. Health Aff (Millwood) 2005;24(3):843–53.
8. Glossary of times used for scheduling and monitoring diagnostic and therapeutic procedures. AORN J 1997;66(4):601–6.
9. Available at: http://www.aqihq.org/AQISchDoc/default.html. Accessed July 25, 2010.
10. Walsh J, Hurrell M, Wu H, et al. Available at: http://www.asaabstracts.com/strands/asaabstracts/abstract.htm;jsessionid=0a5051c416f8eda5357d4bf6f28b561?year=2009&index=8&absnum=1564. Accessed June 4, 2010.
11. Epstein RH, Vigoda MM, Feinstein DM. Anesthesia information management systems: a survey of current implementation policies and practices. Anesth Analg 2007;105:405–11.
12. Egger Halbeis CB, Epstein RH, Macario A, et al. Adoption of anesthesia information management systems by academic departments in the United States. Anesth Analg 2008;107:1323–9.
13. Weiss YG, Cotev S, Drenger B, et al. Patient data management systems in anaesthesia: an emerging technology. Can J Anaesth 1995;42:914–21.
14. Egger Halbeis CB, Epstein RH. The value proposition of anesthesia information management systems. Anesthesiol Clin 2008;26:665–79.
15. Hamilton WK. Will we see automated record keeping systems in common use in anesthesia during our lifetime? The automated anesthetic record is inevitable and valuable. J Clin Monit 1990;6:333–4.
16. Bloomfield EL, Feinglass NG. The anesthesia information management system for electronic documentation: what are we waiting for? J Anesth 2008;22:404–11.
17. O'Sullivan CT, Dexter F, Lubarsky DA, et al. Evidence-based management assessment of return on investment from anesthesia information management systems. AANA J 2007;75:43–8.
18. Balust J, Macario A. Can anesthesia information management systems improve quality in the surgical suite? Curr Opin Anaesthesiol 2009;22:215–22.
19. Sandberg WS. Anesthesia information management systems: almost there. Anesth Analg 2008;107:1100–2.
20. Muravchick S, Caldwell JE, Epstein RH, et al. Anesthesia information management system implementation: a practical guide. Anesth Analg 2008;107:1598–608.
21. Muravchick S. Anesthesia information management systems. Curr Opin Anaesthesiol 2009;22:764–8.
22. Benson M, Junger A, Fuchs C, et al. Using an anesthesia information management system to prove a deficit in voluntary reporting of adverse events in a quality assurance program. J Clin Monit Comput 2000;16:211–7.
23. Brenck F, Hartmann B, Katzer C, et al. Hypotension after spinal anesthesia for cesarean section: identification of risk factors using an anesthesia information management system. J Clin Monit Comput 2009;23:85–92.
24. Dexter F, Bayman EO, Epstein RH. Statistical modeling of average and variability of time to extubation for meta-analysis comparing desflurane to sevoflurane. Anesth Analg 2010;110:570–80.
25. Epstein RH, Gratch DM, Grunwald Z. Development of a scheduled drug diversion surveillance system based on an analysis of atypical drug transactions. Anesth Analg 2007;105:1053–60.

26. Sanborn KV, Castro J, Kuroda M, et al. Detection of intraoperative incidents by electronic scanning of computerized anesthesia records. Comparison with voluntary reporting. Anesthesiology 1996;85:977–87.

27. Junger A, Hartmann B, Benson M, et al. The use of an anesthesia information management system for prediction of antiemetic rescue treatment at the postanesthesia care unit. Anesth Analg 2001;92:1203–9.

28. Rohrig R, Hartmann B, Junger A, et al. Corrected incidences of co-morbidities - a statistical approach for risk-assessment in anesthesia using an AIMS. J Clin Monit Comput 2007;21:159–66.

29. Vigoda MM, Rodriguez LI, Wu E, et al. The use of an anesthesia information system to identify and trend gender disparities in outpatient medical management of patients with coronary artery disease. Anesth Analg 2008;107:185–92.

30. Dexter F, Penning DH, Lubarsky DA, et al. Use of an automated anesthesia information system to determine reference limits for vital signs during cesarean section. J Clin Monit Comput 1998;14:491–8.

31. Epstein RH, Dexter F, Piotrowski E. Automated correction of room location errors in anesthesia information management systems. Anesth Analg 2008;107:965–71.

32. Kheterpal S, Gupta R, Blum JM, et al. Electronic reminders improve procedure documentation compliance and professional fee reimbursement. Anesth Analg 2007;104:592–7.

33. Eden A, Pizov R, Toderis L, et al. The impact of an electronic reminder on the use of alarms after separation from cardiopulmonary bypass. Anesth Analg 2009;108: 1203–8.

34. Dexter F, Epstein RH, Lee JD, et al. Automatic updating of times remaining in surgical cases using bayesian analysis of historical case duration data and "instant messaging" updates from anesthesia providers. Anesth Analg 2009;108:929–40.

35. Sandberg WS, Sandberg EH, Seim AR, et al. Real-time checking of electronic anesthesia records for documentation errors and automatically text messaging clinicians improves quality of documentation. Anesth Analg 2008;106:192–201.

36. Fuchs C, Quinzio L, Benson M, et al. Integration of a handheld based anaesthesia rounding system into an anaesthesia information management system. Int J Med Inf 2006;75:553–63.

37. Epstein RH, Ekbatani A, Kaplan J, et al. Development of a staff recall system for mass casualty incidents using cell phone text messaging. Anesth Analg 2010; 110:871–8.

38. Spring SF, Sandberg WS, Anupama S, et al. Automated documentation error detection and notification improves anesthesia billing performance. Anesthesiology 2007;106:157–63.

39. Lee YL, Wu JL, Wu HS, et al. The use of portable computer for information acquirement during anesthesiologist's ward round in acute pain service. Acta Anaesthesiol Taiwan: Official Journal of the Taiwan Society of Anesthesiologists 2007;45:79–87.

40. Vigoda MM, Gencorelli F, Lubarsky DA. Changing medical group behaviors: increasing the rate of documentation of quality assurance events using an anesthesia information system. Anesth Analg 2006;103:390–5.

41. O'Reilly M, Talsma A, VanRiper S, et al. An anesthesia information system designed to provide physician-specific feedback improves timely administration of prophylactic antibiotics. Anesth Analg 2006;103:908–12.

42. Wax DB, Beilin Y, Levin M, et al. The effect of an interactive visual reminder in an anesthesia information management system on timeliness of prophylactic antibiotic administration. Anesth Analg 2007;104:1462–6.

43. Driscoll WD, Columbia MA, Peterfreund RA. An observational study of anesthesia record completeness using an anesthesia information management system. Anesth Analg 2007;104:1454–61.
44. Vigoda MM, Gencorelli FJ, Lubarsky DA. Discrepancies in medication entries between anesthetic and pharmacy records using electronic databases. Anesth Analg 2007;105:1061–5.
45. Wax D, Neustein S. Watch your back. J Clin Monit Comput 2009;23:187–8.
46. Vigoda MM, Lubarsky DA. Failure to recognize loss of incoming data in an anesthesia record-keeping system may have increased medical liability. Anesth Analg 2006;102:1798–802.
47. Vigoda MM, Lubarsky DA. The medicolegal importance of enhancing timeliness of documentation when using an anesthesia information system and the response to automated feedback in an academic practice. Anesth Analg 2006;103:131–6.
48. Dutton RP, Stansbury LG, Leone S, et al. Trauma mortality in mature trauma systems: are we doing better? An analysis of trauma mortality patterns, 1997–2008. J Trauma 2010;69(3):620–6.
49. Vila H, Soto R, Cantor AB, et al. Comparative outcomes analysis of procedures performed in physician offices and ambulatory surgery centers. Arch Surg 2003;138:991–5.

Integration of the Enterprise Electronic Health Record and Anesthesia Information Management Systems

Scott R. Springman, MD

KEYWORDS

• Informatics • Anesthesia • Quality

By 2010 26% of hospitals reported having some form of AIMS. In 2010 63% of hospitals with only surgery-related information systems planned on buying an AIMS.[1] Though small, the market for anesthesia information management systems (AIMS) is growing at 15% to 20% per year. Even this may be an underestimation after recent legislation intended to expand electronic health documentation. Of note, many AIMS have been developed with a focus only on the unique needs of anesthesia providers, and are not fully integrated into other electronic health record (EHR) components of the *entire* affiliated hospital and/or ambulatory medical system (herein called the "enterprise"). The goal of this article is to explore current developments in the push to expand enterprise health information technology (HIT), and the pros and cons of full enterprise integration with an AIMS.

Enterprise HIT should provide comprehensive management of medical information and secure information exchange between providers, as well as health care consumers and providers. The expanded use of HIT has the potential to improve quality medical care, reduce medical errors, increase the efficiency of care, reduce unnecessary health care costs, reduce administrative inefficiencies, decrease paperwork, expand access to affordable care, and improve the health of the general population.

Since the publication of the Institute or Medicine (IOM) 1999 report "To Err is Human"[2] and the subsequent follow-up reports "Crossing the Quality Chasm"[3] (2001) and "Patient Safety, Achieving A New Standard of Care"[4] (2003), a recurring suggestion to improve safety has been the promulgation of HIT. HIT has regularly

Financial Disclosure: The author has nothing to disclose.
Funding Support: None.
Anesthesiology Department, University of Wisconsin School of Medicine and Public Health, 600 Highland Avenue, Madison, WI 53792, USA
E-mail address: srspring@wisc.edu

Anesthesiology Clin 29 (2011) 455–483
doi:10.1016/j.anclin.2011.05.007
1932-2275/11/$ – see front matter © 2011 Elsevier Inc. All rights reserved.

been touted as a way to meet the 6 aims of the IOM: safety, efficiency, timeliness, efficacy, patient-centeredness, and equitability.

To understand why anesthesia providers should embrace HIT on a health system–wide basis, one must review recent HIT history and review HIT concepts. The list of HIT terms and acronyms can be confusing, especially because not everyone uses them the same way. A personal health record (PHR) is a *patient-based* record that includes health care information from all sources; this may be portable or web-based. An electronic document system (EDS) is *provider-based* and simply records information electronically, either as scanned images or as electronically entered text or dictation. An EHR connotes capability considerably above that of a simple EDS. An EHR is a provider-based record that encompasses all enterprise-wide health documentation for a patient. An EHR may be called an "enterprise electronic medical record," or alternately a "comprehensive" EMR, or sometimes simply an EMR. This article uses the term EHR, except if other investigators explicitly use another.

The EHR has been defined as a longitudinal electronic record of patient health information generated by one or more encounters in any care delivery setting. This information includes (but is not restricted to) patient demographics, provider documentation (progress notes, nursing notes, reports, flowcharts, and so forth), problem lists, medications, vital signs, past medical, surgical, or social history, immunizations, electronic picture archiving and communication systems (PACS), laboratory data, and radiology text reports. The EHR should automate and streamline the clinician's workflow, although this is easier said than done. The EHR has the ability to generate a complete record of a clinical patient encounter as well as supporting other electronic care-related activities, either directly or indirectly, via interfaces. Going beyond the basics, advanced comprehensive support includes evidence-based clinical decision support (CDS), quality management, and outcomes reporting.[5] **Table 1** shows some characteristics of basic versus comprehensive (enterprise) EHRs.

EHRs should, in theory, provide instantaneous access to the entirety of the patient's health information to create better health care decisions, improve communication and coordination of acute care, and provide information for better long-term chronic and preventative care. **Box 1** lists reasons why the Centers for Medicare and Medicaid Services (CMS) believe that EHRs are better than paper.

President Obama, addressing the Joint Session of Congress in February 2009, said "our recovery plan will invest in electronic health records and new technology that will reduce errors, bring down costs, ensure privacy, and save lives."

He referred, of course, to the Health Information Technology for Economic and Clinical Health (HITECH) Act, under the 2009 American Recovery and Reinvestment Act (ARRA), which gives the US Department of Health and Human Services (HHS) the authority to establish a set of programs, incentives, and penalties for adoption and use of certified EHR systems.[6] The stated goal of this initiative is to improve the quality, safety, and efficiency of health care.[7] The Act's Final Rule also includes standards for content, vocabulary, transmission, security, and quality.

Before 2015, the HITECH Act offers Medicare incentive payments for hospitals and providers that can implement a "certified" EHR system and meet a set of so-called Meaningful Use (MU) requirements of certified EHR systems. MU is a set of implementation and standards to be enforced by the ARRA, and this is in addition to existing Health Insurance Portability and Accountability Act (HIPAA) standards and regulations. Through HITECH, the federal government will support the adoption and use of EHRs. Supporting incentive payments to providers may total up to $27 billion over 10 years, or up to $44,000 (through Medicare) and $63,750 (through Medicaid) per clinician. The HITECH Act also enacts a 2015 deadline for hospitals and physician

Table 1
Electronic requirements for classification of hospitals as having a comprehensive or basic electronic records system[a]

Requirement	Comprehensive EHR System	Basic EHR System with Clinician Notes	Basic EHR System Without Clinician Notes
Clinical Documentation			
Demographic characteristics of patients	√	√	√
Physicians' notes	√	√	
Nursing assessments	√	√	
Problem lists	√	√	√
Medication lists	√	√	√
Discharge summaries	√	√	√
Advance directives	√		
Testing and Imaging Results			
Laboratory reports	√	√	√
Radiologic reports	√	√	√
Radiologic images	√		
Diagnostic test results	√	√	√
Diagnostic test images	√		
Consultant reports	√		
Computerized Provider Order Entry			
Laboratory tests	√		
Radiologic tests	√		
Medications	√	√	√
Consultation requests	√		
Nursing orders	√		
Decision Support			
Clinical guidelines	√		
Clinical reminders	√		
Drug-allergy alerts	√		
Drug-drug interaction alerts	√		
Drug-laboratory interaction alerts (eg, digoxin and low level of serum potassium)	√		
Drug-dose support (eg, renal dose guidance)	√		
Adoption level – % hospitals (95% confidence interval)	1.5 (1.1–2.0)	7.6 (6.8–8.1)	10.9 (9.7–12.0)

[a] A comprehensive electronic health records (EHR) system is defined as a system with electronic functionalities in all clinical units. A basic electronic records system is defined as a system with electronic functionalities in at least one clinical unit.

Box 1
Electronic health records improve care by enabling functions that paper records cannot deliver

EHRs can make a patient's health information available when and where it is needed—it is not locked away in one office or another

EHRs can bring a patient's total health information together in one place, and always be current—clinicians need not worry about not knowing the drugs or treatments prescribed by another provider, so care is better coordinated

EHRs can support better follow-up information for patients—for example, after a clinical visit or hospital stay, instructions and information for the patient can be effortlessly provided; and reminders for other follow-up care can be sent easily or even automatically to the patient

EHRs can improve patient and provider convenience—patients can have their prescriptions ordered and ready even before they leave the provider's office, and insurance claims can be filed immediately from the provider's office

EHRs can link information with patient computers to point to additional resources—patients can be more informed and involved as EHRs are used to help identify additional web resources

EHRs don't just "contain" or transmit information, they also compute with it—for example, a qualified EHR will not merely contain a record of a patient's medications or allergies, it will also automatically check for problems whenever a new medication is prescribed and alert the clinician to potential conflicts

EHRs can improve safety through their capacity to bring all of a patient's information together and automatically identify potential safety issues—providing "decision support" capability to assist clinicians

EHRs can deliver more information in more directions, while reducing "paperwork" time for providers—for example, EHRs can be programmed for easy or automatic delivery of information that needs to be shared with public health agencies or quality measurement, saving clinician time

EHRs can improve privacy and security—with proper training and effective policies, electronic records can be more secure than paper

EHRs can reduce costs through reduced paperwork, improved safety, reduced duplication of testing, and most of all improved health through the delivery of more effective health care

From Center for Medicare and Medicaid Services. Electronic health records at a glance 2010. Available at: http://www.hss.state.ak.us/hit/docs/FactSheet_EHR.pdf.

---

offices to meet these requirements in order to avoid subsequent Medicare payment penalties.[7–10]

CMS has proposed MU requirements in each of 5 areas[10]:

- Improve quality, safety, and efficiency, and reduce health disparities
- Engage patients and families in their health care
- Improve care coordination
- Improve population and public health
- Ensure adequate privacy and security of health information.

An Eligible Provider and an Eligible Hospital shall be considered a "meaningful EHR user" during an EHR reporting period for a payment year if they meet 3 requirements. First, the provider uses a "qualified" and "certified" EHR in a "meaningful" manner (eg, computerized practitioner order entry [CPOE], e-Prescribing, Barcode medication administration). Second, the provider uses certified EHR technology that provides for the electronic exchange of health information to improve the quality of health care through care coordination. Finally, clinical quality measures and other measures are submitted to government-approved agencies in a manner dictated by the HHS Secretary.

The published Final Rule for the EHR Incentive Program states that: "Qualified EHR" means an electronic record of health-related information on an individual that: (1) includes patient demographic and clinical health information, such as medical history and problem lists; and (2) has the capacity: (a) to provide CDS; (b) to support physician order entry; (c) to capture and query information relevant to health care quality; and (d) to exchange electronic health information with, and integrate such information from other sources.[6]

The Final Rule divides full requirements into a "Core" set, plus an additional "Menu" set of functionality from which providers may choose 5 of 10 items.[6] This "2-track" approach ensures that the basic elements of meaningful EHR use will be met by all providers qualifying for incentive payments, and yet still allows some flexibility. **Box 2** lists the Core set and **Box 3** the Menu set. The overall requirements advance over time in 3 stages: stage 1: capture and share clinical data; stage 2: provide advanced clinical processes with CDS; stage 3: achieve improved outcomes.

Congress specified 3 types of requirements for MU: (1) use of certified EHR technology in a "meaningful" manner (for example, electronic prescribing); (2) that the certified EHR technology is connected in a manner that provides for the electronic exchange of health information to improve the quality of care; and (3) that, in using certified EHR technology, the provider submits to the Secretary information on clinical quality measures and such other measures selected by the Secretary.

Among the MU requirements is improved communication among providers and patients, so that each can send data to the other for referral and care coordination. Providers can send alerts and reminders to patients as well as permitting patients

---

Box 2
HITECH Core set (14 items for providers, 15 for hospitals)

Record patient demographics, preliminary cause of death in the event of mortality

Record vital signs and chart changes

Maintain up-to-date problem list of current and active diagnoses

Maintain active medication list

Maintain active medication allergy list

Record smoking status

Provide patients with clinical summaries

Provide patients with an electronic copy of their health record

Transmit permissible prescriptions electronically

CPOE for medication orders

Implement drug-drug and drug-allergy interaction checks

Implement capability to electronically exchange key clinical information among providers and patient-authorized entities

Implement one CDS rule and ability to track compliance with the rule

Implement systems to protect privacy and security of patient data in the EHR

Report clinical quality measures to CMS or states

Box 3
HITECH Menu set (requires 5/10 choices)

Implement drug formulary checks

Incorporate clinical laboratory test results into EHRs as structured data

Generate lists of patients by specific conditions to use for quality improvement, reduction of disparities, research, or outreach

Use EHR technology to identify patient-specific education resources and provide those to the patient as appropriate

Perform medication reconciliation between care settings

Provide summary of care record for patients referred or transitioned to another provider or setting

Submit electronic immunization data to immunization registries or immunization information systems

Submit electronic syndromic surveillance data to public health agencies

Record advance directives for patients 65 years of age or older

Submit of electronic data on reportable laboratory results to public health agencies

Send reminders to patients (per patient preference) for preventive and follow-up care

Provide patients with timely electronic access to their health information (including laboratory results, problem list, medication lists, medication allergies)

---

to view their own medical records. The medical organization is additionally obliged to give clinical summaries to patients and send quality data to CMS.

Eight of 10 hospital chief information officers (CIOs) recently surveyed by PriceWaterhouseCoopers LLP said they are concerned or very concerned that they will not be able to demonstrate MU of EHRs within the federally established deadline of 2015. Nonetheless, they believe that MU will drive and accelerate adoption of EHRs.[11] In an August 2010 survey of members of the College of Health Information Management Executives (CHIME), 38% of CIO respondents from academic medical centers expect to qualify for stimulus funding within the first 6 months, compared with only 22% of CIOs at community hospitals. In general, executives of larger organizations say they are more likely to qualify for funding within 6 months, as compared with responses from smaller organizations.[12]

EHR CERTIFICATION

The independent Certification Commission for Healthcare Information Technology (CCHIT) is a federally recognized certification body for EHRs. Through the new HITECH certification program, additional certification bodies will be established to test and certify EHR technology.[13] The federal Office of the National Coordinator (ONC) is establishing incentive programs standards, implementation specifications, and certification criteria for HIT. Working with ONC, the National Institute of Standards and Technology (NIST) is developing the functional and conformance testing requirements, test cases, and test tools for the proposed Health HIT certification programs.

In a report published in 2009, it was stated that fewer than 2% of United States hospitals had a "comprehensive" electronic records system (ie, present in all clinical units), and an additional 7.6% had only a basic system (ie, present in at least one clinical unit). CPOE was implemented in only 17% of hospitals. Barriers cited to the implementation of an EHR included concerns about capital for purchase (74%) and/or maintenance costs (44%), physician resistance (36%), unclear return on investment (32%), and HIT staff shortages (30%).[14] All factors except physician resistance were cited more frequently by hospitals without an EMR.[14]

At the time of this writing, only 2 HIT products (Eclipsys Corporation and Epic Systems Corporation) had full single-vendor "enterprise-wide" designation from CCHIT. Enterprise-wide is defined as including ambulatory, inpatient, and emergency department systems. The Healthcare Information and Management Systems Society (HIMSS) defines 7 stages in the functionality of EHRs as shown in **Table 2**. In the fall of 2010, there were only 8 health systems that had achieved full "Stage 7."[15]

A 2008 survey estimated that at least 44% of academic anesthesia departments either had implemented or had planned on implementing an AIMS.[16] Even before the HITECH Act, the prediction in 2008 was that there would be a strong upswing in AIMS installations. Despite this, there has been continued skepticism that anesthesia departments would agree to submit to the "yoke" of an enterprise EHR that is not fully customized to anesthesiologists' needs.[17]

BENEFITS OF AN EHR

Enterprise EHR adoption should be an evolution, but to many clinicians it often seems more like a revolution. Adoption of an EHR may be a major upheaval to clinicians' professional lives. EHRs can radically change current documentation method(s), workflows, billing practices, scheduling, patient follow-up methods, communication, and messaging.

No matter what the attitudes of providers, these changes are inevitable. David Blumenthal, until 2011 the director of the government's ONC for Health Information Technology, has said "the use of health information technology will be regarded as a core technical competence for (Health) professionals."[18] Dr Farzad Mostashari assumed the directorship in 2011 and continues to carry on the work of implementing the HiTech Act.

It can be argued that the evidence of a favorable benefit to the general use of EHRs is inconclusive from a scientifically proven standpoint, but leaders in the field of patient safety strongly believe that the benefits are, indeed, real.[19–21] **Table 3** lists many of the oft-cited benefits.

Proposed EHR advantages include increased efficiencies related to administrative tasks, allowing for more interaction with and information transfer to patients, caregivers, and clinical care coordinators. Monitoring of patient care could be improved because EHR systems electronically display results from laboratory tests, radiology procedures, and other diagnostic examinations so that providers can immediately access information. CPOE can reduce mistakes caused by illegible handwriting and delays in filling orders, or eliminate lost orders. Automatic reminders and prompts can improve preventive care, diagnosis, treatment, and chronic disease management.

Most would argue that EHRs do have real benefits. However, there is some disagreement about exactly who benefits most. Providers may benefit considerably from enhanced access to legible health records, but the trade-off for them is an increased burden of record-keeping and data entry. Providers also may be forced into unfamiliar and more difficult workflows. Patients may receive care that is better documented, coordinated, and monitored, but it may be at the expense of providers seemingly paying more attention to the computer monitor than to them. Health

Table 2		
Seven stages in the functionality of EHRs and recent health care adoption of stages		
HIMSS Stage and Capabilities	**2010 Q 1 (%)**	**2010 Q 2 (%)**
Stage 0: The organization has not installed all of the key ancillary department systems (eg, laboratory, pharmacy, radiology)	11.4	11.2
Stage 1: Major ancillary clinical systems are installed (ie, pharmacy, laboratory, radiology)	6.9	6.8
Stage 2: Major ancillary clinical systems feed data to a clinical data repository (CDR) that provides physician access for retrieving and reviewing results. The CDR contains a controlled medical vocabulary, and the clinical decision support/rules engine (CDS) for rudimentary conflict checking. Information from document imaging systems may be linked to the CDR at this stage. The hospital is HIE capable at this stage and can share whatever information it has in the CDR with other patient care stakeholders	16.5	15.5
Stage 3: Nursing/clinical documentation (eg, vital signs, flow sheets) is required; nursing notes, care plan charting, and/or the electronic medication administration record (eMAR) system are scored with extra points, and are implemented and integrated with the CDR for at least one service in the hospital. The first level of clinical decision support is implemented to conduct error checking with order entry (ie, drug/drug, drug/food, drug/laboratory conflict checking normally found in the pharmacy). Some level of medical image access from PACS is available for access by physicians outside the Radiology department via the organization's intranet	50	50.2
Stage 4: CPOE for use by any clinician is added to the nursing and CDR environment along with the second level of clinical decision support capabilities related to evidence-based medicine protocols. If one patient service area has implemented CPOE with physicians entering orders and has completed the previous stages, then this stage has been achieved	7.7	9.7
Stage 5: The closed-loop medication administration environment is fully implemented. The eMAR and bar coding or other auto-identification technology, such as radiofrequency identification (RFID), are implemented and integrated with CPOE and pharmacy to maximize point-of-care patient safety processes for medication administration	5	3.2
Stage 6: Full physician documentation/charting (structured templates) is implemented for at least one patient care service area. Level 3 of clinical decision support provides guidance for all clinician activities related to protocols and outcomes in the form of variance and compliance alerts. A full complement of PACS systems provides medical images to physicians via an intranet and displaces all film-based images	1.8	2.6
Stage 7: The hospital no longer uses paper charts to deliver and manage patient care and has a mixture of discrete data, document images, and medical images within its EMR environment. Clinical data warehouses are being used to analyze patterns of clinical data to improve quality of care and patient safety. Clinical information can be readily shared via standardized electronic transactions (ie, CCD) with all entities who are authorized to treat the patient, or a health information exchange (ie, other nonassociated hospitals, ambulatory clinics, subacute environments, employers, payers, and patients in a data-sharing environment). The hospital demonstrates summary data continuity for all hospital services (eg, inpatient, outpatient, emergency department, and with any owned or managed ambulatory clinics)	0.7	0.8

From HIMSS. Stage 7 hospitals. 2010. Available at: http://www.himssanalytics.org/hc_providers/stage7Hospitals.asp. Accessed June 28, 2011; with permission.

Table 3
Cited benefits of EHRs

Role for Electronic Documentation	Goals and Features of Redesigned Systems
Providing access to information	Ensure ease, speed, and selectivity of information searches; aid cognition through aggregation, trending, contextual relevance, and minimizing superfluous data
Recording and sharing assessments	Provide a space for recording thoughtful, succinct assessments, differential diagnoses, contingencies, and unanswered questions, facilitate sharing and review of assessments by both patients and other clinicians
Maintain dynamic patient history	Carry forward information for recall, avoiding repetitive patient querying and recording while minimizing copying and pasting
Maintaining problem lists	Ensure that problem lists are integrated into workflow to allow for continuous updating
Tracking medications	Record medications that patient is actually taking, patient response to medications, and adverse effects to avert misdiagnoses and ensure timely recognition of medication problems
Tracking tests	Integrate management of diagnostic test results into note workflow to facilitate review, assessment, and responsive action as well as documentation of these steps
Ensuring coordination and continuity	Aggregate and integrate data from all care episodes and fragmented encounters to permit thoughtful decisions
Enabling follow-up	Facilitate patient education about potential red-flag conditions; track follow-up
Providing feedback	Automatically provide feedback to clinicians upstream, facilitating learning from outcomes of diagnostic decisions
Providing prompts	Provide checklists to minimize reliance on memory and directed questioning to aid in diagnostic thoroughness and problem solving
Providing placeholder for resumption of work	Delineate clearly in the record where clinicians should resume work after interruption, preventing lapses in data collection and thought process
Calculating Bayesian probabilities	Embed calculator into notes to reduce errors and minimize biases in subjective estimation of diagnostic probabilities
Providing access to information sources	Provide instant access to knowledge resource through context-specific "infobuttons" triggered by keywords in notes that link user to relevant textbooks and guidelines
Offering second opinion or consultation	Integrate immediate online or telephone access to consultants to answer questions related to referral triage, testing strategies, or definitive diagnostic assessments
Increasing efficiency	More thoughtful design, workflow integration, and distribution of documentation burden could speed up charting, freeing time for communication and cognition

From Schiff GD, Bates DW. Can electronic clinical documentation help prevent diagnostic errors? N Engl J Med 2010;362(12):1067.

systems reap a windfall from better access to data for managing both patients and providers, but the immense initial cost of personnel, software, and hardware must be considered. Moreover, the initial cost does not end after the system goes live. The costs of HIT support continue forever.

Although many anesthesia providers have had a long-standing wish to implement an AIMS, significant challenges have been recognized for many years.[22] Despite this, because of the HITECH Act it is certain that the pace of AIMS adoption will accelerate. Beyond the benefit of meeting government mandates, there is little doubt that, at the least, using an AIMS there is better physiologic data-recording accuracy in anesthesia care.[23-25] Recent excellent recommendations for AIMS functionality have been published by Muravchick and colleagues,[26] and include thoughtful questions that must be addressed by each organization when choosing or customizing an AIMS.

The challenges facing anesthesia providers when the health system implements a plan for an enterprise EHR vary, depending on their previous experience with AIMS. The possible scenarios range from providers having no previous clinical EHR experience to providers working with a full AIMS already in place.

- Scenario 1: Anesthesia service uses paper documentation now, but will transition to a stand-alone AIMS, without a full EHR.
- Scenario 2: Anesthesia service uses paper documentation now, but will transition to full EHR with the EHR's own integrated AIMS module.
- Scenario 3: Anesthesia service uses or plans a stand-alone AIMS now, but will transition to a full EHR, and retain the original stand-alone AIMS module.
- Scenario 4: Anesthesia service uses a stand-alone AIMS now, but will transition to a full EHR, and switch to the EHR's own AIMS module.

Although Scenario 1 has been more common in the past, it is unlikely to be repeated much in the new, government-regulated health-IT world we find ourselves in. With the passage of recent legislation, the question is not whether every health care system *will* have a full enterprise EHR, it is only *when* it will occur. If the advantages of increased coordination of care, instantaneous access to up-to-date and accurate information, and CDS (among others) were not enough by themselves, the new financial incentives make enterprise and integrated systems inevitable.

It is easier to understand why an anesthesia service would move from paper to an AIMS than it is to see why it would move from an already satisfactory AIMS to a completely different AIMS, even if it is tightly integrated with its own enterprise EHR. Staying with an existing stand-alone AIMS that is not part of an enterprise product (Scenario 3) is sometimes an option, but significant initial and ongoing interface development must occur so that both the enterprise EHR and the AIMS can continuously communicate. It is likely very tempting for anesthesia providers to stay with a known user interface in a mature product rather than migrating to one that will undoubtedly have development growing pains. Providers often would rather not be required to change to a different system that is not as customized as they are used to, or deal with a totally different interface "look and feel," as well as learning changed workflows. However, the initial convenience to the anesthesia providers for retaining the status quo must be balanced against the long-term headaches of maintaining a working interface with the rest of the EHR. Sometimes, reluctantly, there is simply no choice for the anesthesia service. The medical center organization may have decided that the benefits of a fully integrated EHR far outweigh the wishes of individual clinical services to retain their own "best of breed" HIT products. Local political forces may force the decision and be the major factor.

Likewise, although the organization could take many different stand-alone specialty-specific EHR products from multiple vendors and join them together like electronic jigsaw-puzzle pieces, there is major (and sometimes just unacceptable) HIT overhead involved in making and keeping all modules integrated and functional.

There is the possibility that future advances may be made in "cloud computing," free advertisement-supported EHR applications, or master systems that could integrate many separate applications together. It remains to be seen whether these could effectively compete with a single-vendor EHR.

CONCERNS ABOUT SAFETY AND USABILITY OF EHRs

An EHR is a useful tool, but it is not a magic wand or a panacea. Like all tools, it can have flaws and be misused, and it can even cause errors and patient harm.[27] This potential harm to patients has been termed "e-iatrogenesis," and the rush to roll out EHRs has not always taken this potential danger into account.[28] EHRs improve the legibility of and access to information. However, depending on design, EHRs may not improve appropriate use or providers' understanding of available information. It is critical that clinicians are continuously engaged in developing the systems and related work flows inherent in the use of an AIMS, as well as the entire enterprise EHR. Wachter put it succinctly: "…it will be important for clinicians, health care organizations, regulators, payers, and vendors to collectively appreciate the negative consequences of poorly designed systems and rapidly improve the systems to minimize any transitional harm."[29]

Not everyone believes that the advantages of an EHR outweigh potential problems. Issues include the EHR distracting physicians from the patient, discouraging independent data gathering and assessment, and perpetuating errors.[30] A recent survey found that almost 50% of health care professionals are unsatisfied with the performance of their clinical information systems. Those that were satisfied often settled for less than acceptable system response times.[31] Investigators and clinicians have raised serious concerns about the safety and usability of EHRs in general. This concern is distinct from any Luddite reluctance to accept new technology or change. Users typically have major concerns about how EHRs will affect patient safety and outcomes, as well as their own productivity. Users are often embarrassed to ask for help when first using the EHR. To allow for adjustment to new workflows and incremental changes, many have suggested that the enterprise EHR be delivered step-wise to allow for needed "improvisation" in "adapting and adopting."[32] A good reference on change management in EHR adoption is available.[33]

Campbell and colleagues[34,35] grouped unintended adverse consequences in EHRs/CPOE into 9 categories (in order of decreasing frequency): (1) more/new work for clinicians; (2) unfavorable workflow issues; (3) never-ending system demands; (4) problems related to paper persistence; (5) untoward changes in communication patterns and practices; (6) negative emotions; (7) generation of new kinds of errors; (8) unexpected changes in the power structure; and (9) overdependence on the technology. The investigators attributed many of these unintended consequences to CDS. Another study on CPOE safety/problems found that clinical work is adversely affected by (1) introducing or exposing human/computer interaction problems, (2) altering the pace, sequencing, and dynamics of clinical activities, (3) providing only partial support for the work activities of all types of clinical personnel, (4) reducing clinical situation awareness, and (5) poorly reflecting organizational policy and procedure.[36]

Many EHR systems fail to provide user-friendly interfaces, due to the lack of systematic consideration of human-centered computing issues. In a usability assessment of the military EHR, Saitwal and colleagues[37] found, among other problems, a large number of total steps to complete common tasks, a high average task execution time, and a large number of mental operations. The investigators proposed that this, and other, EHR user interfaces could be improved by reducing the total number of steps to do tasks and the amount of mental effort required for tasks.

In another study, it was determined that a leading CPOE system often facilitated risks of frequent medication errors. Investigators warned that clinicians and hospitals must attend to errors that these systems cause, in addition to errors that they prevent.[38] Khajouei and Jaspers[39] categorized EHR CPOE design aspects into 6 different groups: (1) timing of alerts, (2) log in/out procedures, (3) pick lists and drop-down menus, (4) clues and guidelines, (5) documentation and data entry options, and (6) screen display and layout. Their review showed that the system configuration has a high impact on ease of system use, task behavior of clinicians in ordering drugs, and medication errors. The Joint Commission has recently focused on EHR problems in a Sentinel Event Alert notice.[40]

In many usability studies, the total time it takes clinicians to do a task is the primary outcome measure. Others have maintained, however, that an assessment of workflow fragmentation, pattern recognition, and data visualization are far better measures of the frustration users experience with interfaces.[41] Other studies and statements have focused on measures of user "workarounds," suggested usability guides, "human factors" methods, and even legal concerns.[42–46] Experts warn that robot-like documentation may detract from clinicians using their own judgment, and personal interaction with patients may suffer. If not emphasized, "thinking medicine" may be crushed by an EHR.[30] An excellent discussion and warning about EHR's "myths" is contained in the review by Karsch and colleagues[47] of EHR "fallacies and sober realities." A recent 8-dimensional model emphasizes the interactions that determine the "sociotechnical challenges involved in design, development, implementation, use, and evaluation of HIT within complex adaptive health care systems."[48]

Some have suggested that clinicians simply need adjustment time to accept new ways of doing things. However, a problematic interface and workflow cannot be fully compensated for, no matter how long it is used. A study of EHR usability showed that clinicians' experience with bad usability does not improve with time and, in fact, "time does not heal."[49] Indeed, left to their own devices, end users do not eventually figure it out for themselves.[33] There is no doubt that a poor user interface disrupts clinical workflows. Users are often at the mercy of the vendor's development and change schedule, and decisions are often made by administrators or HIT personnel who may lack adequate clinical experience.[50]

In a survey of users' attitudes after implementing an EHR, many users felt that EHR and CPOE worsened performance and made tasks more difficult and complex. Information contained in colleagues' notes, medications on the discharge list, and data from other hospitals was described as difficult to find ("I'm a savvy user and even I find it cumbersome to get the information"). Feelings of frustration, irritation, and resentment are common (eg, "I'm highly resentful of the fact that somebody's using me as a very overqualified typist"). Complaints about general usability limitations were voiced (eg, "This is stupidly designed. This is designed by someone who is not actually taking care of patients").[51] The power to choose the EHR may not always be in the domain of clinicians, but they should insist that organizational leaders consider issues such as those enumerated in **Box 4**.

Astoundingly, HIT vendors currently enjoy a contractual and legal benefit that renders them virtually liability free—a "hold harmless" clause. HIT vendors are not responsible for errors even when their products are implicated in adverse medical events because (according to this doctrine) physicians, nurses, pharmacists, and health care technicians should be able to identify and correct errors produced by software faults.[52]

When one thinks about it, it is strange and alarming that there are not even quality standards or organized reporting of safety issues for EHR products.[53,54] EHR systems

Box 4
Choosing the right EHR: factors affecting the safety of EHRs

Right Hardware or Software: An EHR system must be capable of supporting required clinical activities

Right Content: Right content includes standard medical vocabularies to encode clinical findings and knowledge

Right User Interface: The right user interface allows clinicians to quickly grasp a complex system safely and efficiently

Right Personnel: Trained and knowledgable personnel are essential for safe use

Right Workflow and Communication: Any disruption in workflow or information transfer is fertile ground for error

Right Organizational Characteristics: As with other safety models, a culture of innovation, exploration, and continual improvement are key organizational factors for safe EHR use

Right State and Federal Rules and Regulations: State and federal regulations may act as barriers or facilitators for achieving safe use

Right Monitoring: Certification process is essential but a detailed post-implementation usability inspection process is also needed

Data from Sittig DF, Singh H. Eight rights of safe electronic health record use. JAMA 2009;302:1111–3.

currently are not approved or inspected by any regulatory agency prior to marketing. CCHIT certification may enumerate desired features of the EHR, but it is inadequate to safeguard the quality and integrity of these products. It has been suggested that there be

...at a minimum, a national EHR adverse event investigation board to investigate (1) any Joint Commission reviewable Sentinel Event for which the organization's root cause analysis suggests that the EHR was a major contributing factor; (2) any EHR-related adverse event that affects more than 100 patients; and (3) all unplanned EHR system downtimes that adversely affect patient care, or create potential for an adverse event, and last for more than 24 hours; affect more than 100 patients; are not the direct result of a natural disaster; occur in organizations that have implemented the key components of an EHR (admission/discharge/transfer; clinical results review; clinician order entry, communication, verification; barcode medication verification; picture archiving and communication; clinical documentation; alert notification; access to the local health information exchange); and simultaneously affect at least two of these key EHR components.[55,56]

Some have suggested that the Food and Drug Administration (FDA) should apply its traditional regulatory framework to EHRs, and require EHR vendors to meet all the same regulatory requirements as other, more traditional devices, including risk-based premarket review. The legal profession is beginning to focus on and argue for increased regulation and oversight of EHRs.[46]

Members of the FDA have even suggested caution. During panel testimony Jeffrey Shuren, Director of FDA's Center for Devices and Radiological Health, stated that EHR problems have included:

- Errors of commission, such as accessing the wrong patient's record or over-writing one patient's information with another's (this sometimes can be an issue in incidents involving medical identity theft)

- Errors of omission or transmission, such as the loss or corruption of vital patient data
- Errors in data analysis, including medication dosing errors of several orders of magnitude
- Incompatibility between multivendor software applications and systems, which can lead to any of the above.[57]

In a recent letter to David Blumenthal, the Department of Health and Hospitals National Coordinator for Health Information Technology, the governmental Health HIT Policy Committee[58] recommended:

A national, transparent oversight process and information system is proposed, similar to a Patient Safety Organization (PSO), with the following components:

- Capacity to monitor actual and near-miss patient harms and classify those associated with HIT systems
- Confidential reporting with liability protection (eg, whistle-blower protection, confidential disclosure of adverse events)
- Ability to investigate serious incidents potentially associated with HIT
- Provision of standardized data-reporting formats that facilitate analysis and evaluation
- Receive reports from patients, clinicians, vendors, and health care organizations
- A reporting process to cover multiple factors including usability, processes, and training
- Receive reports about all HIT systems
- Receive reports from all software sources (eg, vendors, self-developed, and open source)
- Ability to disseminate information about reported hazards.

ENTERPRISE EHR AFFECTS ANESTHESIA WORKFLOWS

Traditionally, the "silo" of traditional operating room (OR) information flow has been simultaneously an irritating limitation as well as a protective cocoon. There have been limitations to exchanging information among providers, but many of the rules that govern workflow in the rest of the medical system did not always pertain to anesthesia care. Workflows, including CPOE and electronic documentation, have been different for perioperative care. As soon as anesthesia providers venture out from this silo into the tight interconnectedness of an enterprise EHR, there are bound to be changes.

Anesthesia departments have traditionally been wary of "big-box" solutions and have preferred customizable stand-alone AIMS that can be locally configured and allow "plug-in" architecture. The recurring mantra has been: "we are different."[17]

Nonetheless, anesthesia services recognize that the benefits of AIMS include physiologic data recordings, enhanced quality assessment, automatic reporting and outcomes measurement, educational and research opportunities, medicolegal protection, tabulation of services, reduction of costs, management of resource use, and assistance in accreditation compliance (including residency review).[59] Further advantages may include increased anesthesia billing and the capture of anesthesia-related charges via improved hospital coding, opportunities for improved instruction of anesthesia trainees, and better mechanisms for monitoring of diversion of controlled substances.

Further, an enterprise EHR offers the ability to merge anesthesia documentation with nursing, perfusion, and surgeon's documentation. There is the opportunity to interface with infusion pumps and other devices, including perfusion services. In addition to enhancing operating suite anesthesia care, coordination of care in anesthesia services outside the OR, pain management, and critical care can occur. Anesthesia-related drug costs may be reduced. As long as a decade ago, Kheterpal suggested that not only should an AIMS be a record keeper (clinical documentation), but should generate a dataset and should have a positive effect on the quality of care, not merely record it.[60]

A recent estimate by the American Medical Association indicated that 61% of anesthesiologists are sued at some time during their careers.[61] The age breakdown among anesthesiologists for litigation exposure was 13.2% at age less than 40 years, 45.5% at ages 40 to 54 years, and 55.3% at age over 55 years. There has been some concern that an EHR/AIMS could increase risk for medical liability. It appears that while specific issues remain, overall risk may not be adversely affected, or may actually decrease.[62–64] A recent analysis of the liability risks includes recommendations to address general liability concerns.[65] Among other liability concerns, bad habits in electronic documentation may expose providers to billing fraud.[66]

Sharing and Integration

Anesthesia collaboration with HIT in an enterprise EHR means sharing responsibility and decision making for building and enhancing the AIMS. HIT does not have unlimited resources and will likely insist on prioritizing any change requests, and will want to follow the policy-mandated steps in "HIT change management." Validating any changes in several "testing environments" is not unusual. These environments are copies of the live "production" environment, and changes, fixes, and updates are validated to ensure that interactions with other components of the EHR are stable and predictable. This validation means that making changes in the AIMS will be more time consuming and may make it less likely that anesthesia providers get exactly the functionality, interface elements, or workflow that they wish. HIT may not allow an anesthesia clinical provider to directly make changes to the EHR, even if he or she collaborates in development or becomes "certified" in the anesthesia module.

An HIT feature that cannot be overemphasized is data reporting. The ability to generate reports on use, costs, quality-indicator trends, and other factors is so critical in today's data-driven world that it is essential to demand sufficient enterprise resources to produce these in a timely and complete way. Reporting will largely become a centralized service. Being relegated to the back of the line for this is not where anesthesia services wants to be or should be.

On paper or in a basic AIMS, anesthesia providers often document the drug and a mass amount. Sometimes they document a fluid volume and a concentration, but the total amount in the syringe, vial, bottle, bag, and so forth matters little to the administering anesthesia provider. When pharmacy controls the details of the medication records, the form of the drug as well as the administered amount becomes important for hospital tracking purposes. Anesthesia providers are masters of ad hoc medication "mixtures," but the EHR/AIMS may not handle these in a way that makes documentation easy. Because anesthesia medication administration is now part of the medication administration record (MAR), certain rules will apply as to how these medications appear to the rest of the organization.

Issues that were process problems between anesthesia services and other health care organization departments prior to an enterprise EHR often must be finally confronted because they become magnified by integration. There is a definite need to "play nice" with others in the merged world.

While anesthesia providers may have had individual or departmental methods for documentation, the need for universal documentation standards for vascular catheters, airways, case "timing events," and others may cause there to be painful compromises by one or more services. On the positive side, documentation of preadmission medications, home health or long-term care facility information, the inpatient MAR, and intensive care unit flowsheets make anesthesia-specific assessment of patients easier. Sharing, therefore, is not always bad. Access to shared patient status should include knowledge of patients' infection isolation condition, the current physical location of patients, transfusion acceptance, resuscitation wishes, current and trend weight and height, and serious allergies. Electronic whiteboards that show and update critical information that is simultaneously synchronized with the EHR should improve multidisciplinary communication and coordination of care.

Clinical Communication and Documentation

Nothing is easier, faster, or more efficient than *not* documenting. There will be a strong need for extra education for anesthesia providers regarding completion of enterprise EHR tasks and documentation. The need and push for throughput and efficiency in anesthesia care can challenge anesthesia providers to document all elements that are deemed "required" by the organization. In the past (the paper era) the OR was often insulated from many aspects of shared documentation.

Clinical documentation should provide both a snapshot and a timeline history of patient health information that is carried forward and updated, thus showing the evolution of the patient's health status, with safeguards that reduce the chance of perpetuating outdated or inaccurate information.

EHRs are often described as the health system's "information superhighway." A superhighway can increase throughput and improve efficiency, but it may also lead to information gridlock if not used correctly. Health systems often regard EHRs as the Holy Grail of administrative and quality data collection and reporting measure acquisition. Instead of legions of chart abstracters, providers become highly-paid data input tools. If the interface is not optimized for data entry and respectful of provider time and workflow, this will lead to much provider resentment. A truly integrated and organized clinical documentation system will allow each successive level of patient care to take advantage of the previous care and not require duplication of data entry.

A significant advantage of an integrated EHR is the use of a shared lexicon (also known as a dictionary or vocabulary) for data, meaning that medications, adverse reactions, clinical events, questions, diagnoses, problem list, and history items can be standardized.

An up-to-date and accurate problem and history list is a critical part of information sharing and care management in an EHR. The maintenance of a current problem list can be a major task for health systems. A structured vocabulary (eg, International Classification of Diseases—ICD9,[67] Intelligent Medical Objects—IMO[68]) and guidelines for use are important so that a full picture of the patient's medical condition can be considered in determining suitability for a specific anesthesia technique. Each of the several dictionaries has pros and cons. Some were primarily designed for billing (ICD9) whereas others are meant for clinical terms (eg, IMO, Systematized Nomenclature of Medicine-Clinical Terms—SNOMED-CT). In addition, organizations may elect to use ICD9 or IMO for the problem list, but use another dictionary that describes medical, surgical, and diagnostic services (Clinical Procedural Terminology—CPT) for anesthesia and surgical coding.

Events or outcomes during anesthesia care can be coded as clinical terms or clinical modification. Most diagnosis vocabulary vendors have standard terms for issues such as "difficult intubation," but "soft" conditions or history such as "awakens slowly from anesthesia" seldom are included. The Anesthesia Patient Safety Foundation has undertaken a Data Dictionary Task Force effort to coordinate anesthesia-specific vocabulary with SNOMED-CT terms.[69,70] An AIMS should be integrated with the EHR such that coded terms are shared and match. The use of a free text diagnosis does not have the same value to subsequent providers or to the organization if it is to be used for data reporting and quality tracking.

An important part of workflow analysis is determining who enters any handwritten information or paper copies of electronic data into the EHR when patients arrive to anesthesia care from outside the organization (not part of the EHR). If records are scanned, how do providers know that they exist and where they are located in the EHR? When paper persists in the EHR world, what is done with it? Will it always be scanned into image files? Who categorizes the multiple scans that may be generated? The need for, and persistence of paper in EHRs must be examined and addressed. In one study the investigators found 11 categories of paper-based workarounds to the use of the EHR. Paper use was related to: (1) efficiency; (2) knowledge/skill/ease of use; (3) memory; (4) sensorimotor preferences; (5) awareness; (6) task specificity; (7) task complexity; (8) data organization; (9) longitudinal data processes; (10) trust; and (11) security.[71] Sometimes paper helped providers. In other cases, paper use was a workaround to the EHR workflow and introduced potential gaps in documentation. It also produced increased risk for medical error. The human-technology factors leading to increased paper included:

- Cumbersome EHR interface design leading to paper notations to help organize facts
- EHR not well integrated into clinical workflow, leading to paper workarounds
- Visual organization of EHR data incompatible with clinician's mental model.[71]

Even if all information is located in the EHR, it may be unintuitive to find. In the paper world, a nurse's preoperative and postoperative care documentation was at the patient's bedside and providers knew to look at it. In the EHR, this information may be located in various information niches, often unfamiliar to anesthesia providers. During the development phase of the EHR, it is worthwhile for anesthesia providers to be cognizant of nursing documentation workflow. This knowledge will provide an opportunity to automatically pull extracts of nursing data into anesthesia documentation or screen views without the requirement to look in multiple unfamiliar screens of the EHR.

EHRs are not necessarily seamless. Even enterprise systems from a single vendor usually have a modular structure. Every module probably does not handle tasks in exactly in the same way. EHRs that are an amalgam of vendor products are guaranteed to have components that need intercomponent translation or augmentation. A good example of this is "scheduling." The method and structure by which the OR schedules patients may be completely different from that of a clinic or a non-OR procedure area. When patients cross boundaries in their care, these differences must be reconciled. Anesthesia care for a single patient in several hospital locations may end up being duplicated in 2 or more scheduling systems, with the subsequent risk of confusion and documentation errors.

Another potential conflict of purposes is the differing needs of the facility and providers to account for "time." Time is a precious commodity in medicine. Time may be tracked for clinical, efficiency, and administrative purposes, but is also critical for professional and facility billing. The EHR may be recording facility billing time completely differently from the way professional billing tracks the same time. This anomaly should be accounted for in determining how patient location and times are reported. If a patient has continuous anesthesia care, but is transported to several locations during the anesthetic (eg, magnetic resonance imaging, interventional radiology, labor and delivery, the OR), can the EHR account for this transition on one anesthesia record and yet provide the tracking that all these locations require?

Access to archived or legacy system information is important for continuity of care, especially in the first few years after implementing an EHR or changing to a different EHR. A full-featured EHR is likely to have resources and a strategy dedicated to this type of transition.

One bright ray of sunshine for clinical providers, including anesthesia providers, is the ability to access this clinical documentation from anywhere within the organization. No longer should the search for patient records include multiple calls to Medical Records or wandering around clinical units looking for physical charts. Indeed, an exciting feature is the ability to access data from outside the physical confines of the buildings themselves. With proper security measures in place, this could improve preparation and planning for anesthesia care.

Integration and Interoperability

The HIMSS defines these terms:

Integration is the arrangement of an organization's information systems in way that allows them to communicate efficiently and effectively and brings together related parts into a single system.[72]

Interoperability is the ability of several health information systems to work together within and across organizational boundaries to advance the effective delivery of health care for individuals and communities.[72]

A shared EHR opens up the world of documentation on patients, both within the organization (surgical and medical clinics, urgent care visits) and, potentially, care given at other health organizations. The latter functionality is specified in the proposed framework of MU. One avenue for health information exchange (HIE) is CONNECT, which is an open-source software solution that supports HIE, both locally and at the national level. CONNECT uses Nationwide Health Information Network standards and governance to make sure that HIEs are compatible with other exchanges being set up throughout the country.[73] HIEs and other health information data exchanges issues will become "hot items" in the MU race.[74]

Patients may ultimately even have access to some or all of their own medical documentation via the EHR. The OpenNotes Project is an example of almost complete access rights.[75] Anesthesia providers may see the time when the use of patient web portals, clinical messaging, and electronic visits allow patients to view and interact with them in ways never seen before.

Security/Authorization

A secure EHR should function such that agents (users or programs) are allowed to perform actions that have been expressly allowed. All EHR systems should include "audit trails," which consist of chronologic records of a user's access and deletion or modification of data. This trail includes user login, file access, and other actions, including attempted unauthorized access. Together, these are components of processes to ensure system integrity, recoverability, and security. HIPAA and the HITECH Act specifically require these, and other, security measures. Once the AIMS is opened to the enterprise, the risk for patient information and data breeches becomes much larger. Anesthesia services should be familiar with the mechanisms and limitations in assigning security access and clearance to all enterprise members, clinical and nonclinical alike.

Enterprise EHR access from within the organizational internal network (intranet) and from outside (using VPN, CITRIX, and so forth) should be managed formally by the central HIT services. This coordination of security and audit trails is one of the advantages of an enterprise solution. Access from outside the organization is a huge benefit to providers, and can allow important extra time to prepare a plan for anesthesia.

In an integrated enterprise EHR, anesthesia users should be able to log in only once to access information. Single Sign-On (SSO) is a mechanism whereby a single action of user authentication and authorization can permit a provider to access all computers and systems where he or she has access permission, without the need to enter multiple passwords. SSO uses centralized servers for all system authentication purposes to ensure that users are theoretically not required to enter their credentials more than once. In reality, clinical systems often require re-authentication for some sensitive data entry. Examples of the need for higher security include orders function, CMS and other third-party payer "attestations," and staffing confirmation. In an enterprise EHR, the authentication screens look the same, and the same password is used.

Anesthesia is different from most other medical care, in that medications are typically given by the provider that "orders" them. A paper anesthesia record is fairly security "loose." There is loose tracking of who did what and who gave what drugs. In an EHR, however, while intraoperative medications do not usually require an individual order, there may be a behind-the-scenes automatic order generated to meet pharmacy, institutional, or state requirements. Once an anesthesia provider ventures out of the intraoperative environment, however, any order typically requires a discrete user authentication.

CPOE

A key distinction between an AIMS and other HIT systems is the handling of medication orders. In most provider situations, a physician specifies an order and someone else, often a nurse, executes it. In a hospital, many times a pharmacist reviews and modifies provider medication orders. However, in the OR the anesthesiologist both gives and executes the order, and the AIMS must be designed with this in mind. Therefore it should not require too many steps, distract from a focus on the patient, or be cumbersome.

The ordering process in an EHR is arguably one of the most important factors, but it is also the one that clinicians may find frustrating and confusing. It is easy to write paper orders in many different ways to indicate the intent, and humans usually are able to decode the variations. However, electronic ordering is not so forgiving. Specific dose amounts, units, administration routes, and administration instructions are usually required. In addition, the health system may have decided to require background clinical information to assist in the clinical interpretation of, say, an electrocardiogram or radiologic test. Justification for ordering a particular drug or test may also be required to control risk, cost, or simply for tracking purposes.

Only users with ordering "security" (permission) can place general orders, although various levels of ordering security may be granted. Often the organization will require that there be an "ordering" user (the provider who places the order), and an "authorizing" user (the provider who has authority to order). In addition, an ordering "mode" can be used for verbal orders or for orders placed via an approved protocol. To make it more confusing, authorizing users may have different security to authorize medications versus "procedures" (eg, tests, treatments). Sometimes these ordering details can be built into the background, but sometimes these extra steps are required.

While general EHR users typically document and order only via their own username and password "logon," the anesthesia record may have several users documenting under one logon, albeit requiring separate user authentication for certain tasks. Alternatively, some EHRs do not allow ordering (even with user authentication) unless the ordering user is also logged on. To make it even more confusing, this may not apply to intraoperative medication administration, but only to orders outside the OR.

Often, EHRs require a patient status, such as "outpatient" or "inpatient." If the order is placed for the wrong status, it may not be accessible to nurses or pharmacists. Similarly, an order may have a "phase of care" (POC) that might include, among others, preoperative/prior to day of surgery, preoperative/day of surgery, intraoperative, postanesthesia care unit recovery, stage II recovery, and inpatient unit. In this way orders can be "signed and held." If an order is not specified for the correct POC, it may not be noticed and "released" by nursing staff at the appropriate time. Many EHR systems also accommodate "pending" of orders. Pended orders live in a kind of limbo, and can only be seen and activated by the original ordering user.

The issues described may not be the only aspects of ordering that providers need to learn. Others relate to the questions: Where can I "see" other providers' orders? Where can I "see" my own orders? How do I modify or discontinue previous orders? How do I know that the orders were actually performed? Which orders need to be cosigned and how do I access them? How is weight-based medication dosing handled? How can I customize order sets? Do I have read-only or full access to the MAR? These issues are only but a few of those that may confuse the anesthesia provider who moves to an EHR.

CPOE has usually been found to be significantly beneficial in minor ways, but several studies reported actual increases in the rate of duplicate orders and failures to discontinue drugs, often attributed to inappropriate selection from a drop-down menu or an inability to view all active medication orders concurrently.[76]

A by-product of CPOE at the organizational level is improved accountability for controlled medications. Of course, the ability of an AIMS to track all drugs is an advantage to the enterprise, but organizational reporting of controlled drugs is mandated by law. Potential improved monitoring by personnel outside the anesthesia department to prevent diversion of drugs could be a benefit to both providers and patients.

Clinical Decision Support

CDS is software crafted to help clinicians choose among patient care options by matching unique patient characteristics, such as patient conditions, test results, or predictive models, to predetermined rules in order to produce patient analysis or guidance. **Box 5** shows some common elements of CDS building. The rules require careful design, implementation, and ongoing maintenance. CDS has been referred to as an inventory of clinical knowledge management tools and techniques.[77]

Basic CDS usually includes drug-allergy and drug-drug checking, basic dosing guidance, formulary recommendations, and duplicate therapy checking. Advanced CDS may support renal insufficiency and age-based guidance, as well as medication-related laboratory checks. Other drug-disease contraindication and drug-pregnancy recommendations may also be present. Enthusiasm for CDS is building, and is part of the HITECH Act's MU.

The sensitivity and specificity of the alerts will determine CDS's clinical utility. At some point false-positive alerts will cause clinicians to ignore and "click-through" alerts, leading to missed clinical intervention opportunities. The optimal "alerting" strategy for clinicians is often debated.[78]

Despite positive opinions about CDS, confirmatory studies are inconclusive. Shojania and colleagues[79] reported that a review of the Cochrane database found that point-of-care computer reminders generally achieve only small to modest improvements in

---

Box 5
Common elements of CDS

Triggers: The events that cause a decision support rule to be invoked. Examples of triggers include prescribing a drug, ordering a laboratory test, or entering a new problem on the problem list.

Input data: The data elements used by a rule to make inferences. Examples include laboratory results, patient demographics, or the problem list.

Interventions: The possible actions a decision support module can take, such as sending a message to a clinician, showing a guideline, or simply logging that an event took place.

Offered choices: Many decision support events require users of a clinical system to make a choice. For example, a rule that fired because a physician entered an order for a drug to which the patient is allergic might allow the clinician to cancel the new order, choose a safer alternative drug, or override the alert and keep the order as written but provide an explanation.

Data from Wright A, Goldberg H, Hongsermeier T, et al. A description and functional taxonomy of rule-based decision support content at a large integrated delivery network. J Am Med Inform Assoc 2007;14(4):489–96; and Wright A, Sittig DF, Ash JS, et al. Clinical decision support capabilities of commercially-available clinical information systems. J Am Med Inform Assoc 2009;16:637–44.

---

provider behavior; this may be only because the CDS systems are not currently optimized. In 2010 the Leapfrog group[80] reported that a study using Leapfrog's web-based simulation tool indicated that half of the potential clinical problems were not detected until study hospitals modified their systems.

Other issues are also evident. Most CDS systems cannot yet access or interpret free text data entry. Data must be coded from a standardized vocabulary. The lack of uniformity in coding medical conditions presents significant obstacles to computer-based assessment systems. Coding of physician data is extremely complex. Inaccurate or incomplete data may cause poor automated recommendations for care.

There is some evidence that anesthesia-specific CDS can catch general documentation errors.[81] Further opportunities include, at a minimum, checking for malignant hyperthermia history, pseudocholinesterase deficiency, allergies, anticoagulant status, and pregnancy risk. Of interest, Epstein has cautioned that CDS could require Institutional Review Board or FDA approval if the computer itself appears to be determining clinical care.[82]

Noteworthy is that system-wide medication alerts may be problematic for anesthesia providers in the intraoperative setting, because many are not applicable to anesthetists. Anesthesia care often involves giving drugs that have minor mixing incompatibilities via the same intravenous line, or drugs that have drug-related side effects of minimal consequence. The challenge in an EHR will be to customize medication CDS to anesthesia care.

Patient Admission, Discharge, Transfer, and Location, and Outpatient Status

Although the physical location of the patient within the building is the most important piece of a workflow, the electronic location (E-location) of the patient can greatly affect the ability of the provider/user to take care of the patient by entering and manipulating information. This E-location usually determines what is displayed in patient tracking or status boards on monitors or workstations throughout the organization. Users may be limited in workflow if the patient is not properly "admitted" or "located/transferred" to their area. Likewise, a status of inpatient or outpatient may change dramatically what providers "see" on their monitors. Sending or printing of laboratory or radiology requisitions may be affected by this location or status. Electronic order transmittal may not work properly. Due to system-wide decisions, only selected users may be able to change patient location or status. Epstein and colleagues[83] have pointed out implications for anesthesia providers with regard to scheduling and patient location for AIMS function.

One of the advantages of an enterprise EHR is in tracking follow-up with patients. Any required repeat visits or care for patients is made easier by having an electronic list of providers' patients who are still in the facility, or even of patients who have returned home or have moved to a long-term care facility.

Infrastructure, Support, and Downtime

An enterprise patient care system should have a well-developed and well-supported system for storage and access to patient records. The system should include an enterprise infrastructure with secure and adequate network bandwidth, a robust network structure, and well-maintained servers. If an AIMS is integrated with or exists as a module of an EHR, it will share many or all of the benefits of the enterprise hardware. The speed of the network, network topology (linkages and redundancy in map of routers, switches, bridges, servers), storage (static and dynamic), and telecommunications integration (paging, cell phones, mobile access, Wi-Fi, Bluetooth) will all affect the available system features and expansion. Hardware, including use of thin or thick clients, should be reasonably current and durable to allow frustration-less use of the EHR and AIMS. Anesthesia providers should be involved in even the most mundane process of equipment selection, such as computer mice and keyboards.

When proper data flow and communication among the components within the network fails, this is known as "downtime," resulting in a temporary (and hopefully short) interruption in one or more modules and functionality. Downtime may be due to either hardware or software issues. Downtime is either planned or unplanned. Required system maintenance and modification will ultimately produce episodes of downtime. These intervals are usually planned so as to minimize interruption of clinical care, but one services' off-peak time is always another services' peak usage. It must be stressed to the various HIT groups that sufficient warnings to all groups and testing (if possible) before taking down any EHR component is essential. Unplanned downtime is the most stressful situation for clinicians and HIT staff alike. The known possible causes and results of service loss should be determined and documented before implementing an EHR or AIMS. Mitigation and recovery strategies should be fully tested ahead of time. Of course, not all failure situations can be anticipated. A clinical and HIT crisis team should always be available to deal with both small-scale and large-scale loss of EHR function. Power loss, network collapse, and server loss will all occur eventually. Organizations should simply plan for this eventuality. There are many different ways to build "toughness" and resiliency into the system infrastructure. Selection of proper network topography and adequate redundancy will minimize some events. All user areas should have a downtime plan, with access to recent read-only clinical information, at a minimum, on "mirror" servers. Reversion to paper documentation sounds easy, but after using an EHR for even a year, users forget (or never knew) the previous paper workflow. The available paper forms may not be current, or even easy to find. It is preferred to have workflows and systems in place that can continue to collect at least some types of data at the local workstation level, even with full network collapse, and then reload the information. This capability is not always present, however, in many EHRs. After the network outage is over, reloading local information into the network can cause confusion if data are not routed to the correct patient's chart. Also, the overlap period of paper and EHR documentation and orders will be confusing, and could be potentially dangerous to patient care.

Some services, such as anesthesia care, that use data captured from physiologic monitors as part of the workflow may have interruptions or even upstream "logjamming" of data. Depending on the system structure, an enterprise electronic data capture system may increase the risk that data can flow into the wrong patient's record, or into the wrong location in the correct patient's record. Difficulties with the data streaming from monitors may be completely isolated from general network problems and will try the patience of local users. Expecting users to troubleshoot the technical aspects of data acquisition while caring for critically ill patients is unrealistic. Debugging tools that automatically troubleshoot should be developed and made available to both HIT staff and users.

Planned downtime is often used to load fixes or updates into the system. When the AIMS is a part of an overall EHR, these fixes and updates may "break" portions of the AIMS. Integrated testing and verification of proper function should always be done before changes are loaded into the working or "production" environment. Even so, complex interactions between components may not always be predictable. Of note, the preoperative and postoperative part of the AIMS, if a module of a single-vendor EHR, is usually more tightly linked in functionality to the rest of the EHR than it is to the intraoperative anesthesia record.

Determination and tracking of system uptime (the inverse of downtime), peak loading ability, system capacity, recovery from data surges, and overall system reliability is critical to improving HIT's ability to handle challenges.

Finally, all organizations, and their component services, must have a full "disaster" plan that takes into account the total unavailability of the EHR during large-scale utility loss that would result, undoubtedly, in a chaotic clinical situation. Natural disasters or terrorism could easily bring most HIT systems to its knees.

Support, Troubleshooting, Fixes, and Upgrades

It is certain that changes to the EHR and AIMS will be needed after going live. Clinicians tend to identify problems and act quickly. Anesthesia providers, in particular, are used to making changes to care "on the fly" with many iterative tweaks, and will expect that same strategy from HIT. In an enterprise EHR, HIT will generally not work that quick. HIT will want prioritization of changes and expect to set time estimates for all projects. Any proposed changes are usually required to go through a sequence of software testing environments (eg, "Build," "Integrated Testing," "Verify," although each vendor has different terminology). This sequence is intended to reduce the chances that unintended consequences and adverse interactions with other components of the EHR will occur. There will need to be an understanding between both clinicians and HIT regarding appropriate expectations for changes. Otherwise, conflict will occur.

The importance of communication and a good working relationship with the health system CIO, the Clinical Medical and Nursing Information Officers, and HIT in general cannot be overemphasized. The anesthesia service will need support and resources to maintain the AIMS module and ensure its ongoing integration with the enterprise EHR. Continuous software and hardware support is necessary, including regular troubleshooting of data-capture issues.

In a stand-alone AIMS, the local anesthesiologist "expert" may have the ability and permission to make direct changes to the product's interface and functionality. In an integrated EHR product, HIT may balk at that high level of participation. Concerns about control of changes and skepticism about the expertise of a non-IT clinician may be difficult to overcome.

Whereas minor and major upgrades to a stand-alone AIMS may occur at will, an EHR anesthesia module usually must wait for the enterprise EHR change schedule. Periodic updates (including those related to anesthesia) are often pushed out to the EHR in multimodule packages. Occasionally, individual components will be updated separately or other modules of the EHR rolled out distinct from these periodic updates. Special care must be taken to monitor in real time the effect these changes have on the network as a whole since data slowdown or loss has occurred (Jeffrey Zupansic, RT and HIT, Madison, WI, personal communication, September, 2010).

To receive a major upgrade of the anesthesia module, the "base" version of the entire EHR must often be upgraded; this can entail up to several years' wait while HIT plans, builds and, of course, finds the resources to finance the upgrade.

When software or hardware problems occur, a stand-alone AIMS will have a standard debugging process. When an AIMS is part of an enterprise EHR, however, EHR intermodule interactions or in-module "system calls" will eventually generate errors or lock-ups. In an enterprise EHR, the clinical user may be in and out of several layers and modules within a short amount of time, mouse-clicking and keyboarding on multiple screens, thus making the inevitable question from the Help Desk all that more difficult: "What were the last 5 (or 10!) actions you performed before the error occurred?" This situation may considerably slow down the search for the source software anomaly. On the other hand, because enterprise EHR modules share many of the same interface elements and functions, HIT may have a greater sense of urgency to fix a problem that is enterprise-wide.

It is very important to have a collaborative relationship with other clinical departments and with HIT when configuring shared components of the EHR, this being especially critical if the anesthesia department is "late to the table" on EHR decisions. By the nature of the care, decisions previously made by key departments, including pharmacy, nursing, and OR management, may limit what is possible in anesthesia workflows.

The cost of HIT investment in any EHR is considerable, at times almost staggering. After planning, building, and implementation comes the inevitable fixes, updates, and upgrades. Every provider and every department considers their own "issues" to be the most important. No HIT department has unlimited personnel or time. It is the norm that requests for changes go through a formalized prioritization process. All requests that have approximately the same priority usually must join the queue for changes or fixes. Where will the anesthesia department fit in the hierarchy of HIT support and development?

Occasionally an entire health system will "home-grow" its entire EHR. There are undoubtedly some unique challenges in this situation for anesthesia services, but the in-house nature of core development and updates may provide an opportunity for customization beyond that available in any commercial system.

SUMMARY

Anesthesia providers will venture out of their traditional silo of care and begin to interact and integrate with the medical system in an enterprise EHR. It is important for clinicians to understand and be willing to participate in the mandated wave of health care informatics. Interaction with clinical documentation, CPOE, and CDS will challenge our old ways of thinking. Significantly, there remain concerns about the safety and usability of EHRs, but there is no stopping their spread. Anesthesia providers must have the willingness and ability to critically examine and change their workflows to accommodate an AIMS that integrates with an enterprise EHR. It is said that people will change when they have a good reason to change and they desire change, and not before.[51] The rationale for an EHR exists; the desire to adopt it must come from within providers and organizations alike.

REFERENCES

1. Anesthesia Documentation 2011: Slow but Steady Progress. KLAS Research Report 4/27/2011. Avaliable at: http://www.klasresearch.com/. Accessed June 28, 2011.
2. IOM. To err is human: building a safer health system. Washington, DC: Institutes of Medicine; 1999.
3. IOM. Crossing the quality chasm: a new health system for the 21st century Washington, DC: Institutes of Medicine; 2001.
4. IOM. Priority areas for national action: transforming health care quality. Washington, DC: Institutes of Medicine; 2003.
5. HIMSS. EHR definition. 2010. Available at: http://www.himss.org/ASP/topics_ehr.asp. Accessed June 28, 2011.
6. HHS. US Department of Health and Human Services. EHR Incentive Programs. Available at: http://www.cms.gov/EHRIncentivePrograms/. Accessed June 28, 2011.
7. Blumenthal D, Tavenner M. The "Meaningful Use" regulation for electronic health records. N Engl J Med 2010;363(6):501–4.
8. CMS. EHR incentive programs. 2010. Available at: http://www.cms.gov/ehrincentiveprograms/. Accessed June 28, 2011.
9. CMS. Fact sheet: CMS finalizes requirements for the Medicare electronic health records (EHR) incentive program. 2010. Available at: http://www.hss.state.ak.us/hit/docs/FactSheet_EHR.pdf. Accessed June 28, 2011.
10. CMS. Fact sheet: CMS and ONC final regulations define meaningful use and set standards for electronic health record incentive program. 2010. Available at: http://www.cms.gov/apps/media/press/factsheet.asp?Counter=3787. Accessed June 28, 2011.
11. PriceWaterhouseCoopers. Ready or not: On the road to the meaningful use of EHRs and health IT. New York (NY): PriceWaterhouseCooper, LLC; 2010.
12. CHIME. CHIME survey finds healthcare CIOs cautiously optimistic about receiving EHR incentive funding. 2010. Available at: http://www.cio-chime.org/advocacy/CHIMEMUSurveyReport.pdf. Accessed June 28, 2011.
13. ONC. Office of the national coordinator for health information technology—authorized testing and certification bodies. 2010. Available at: http://healthit.hhs.gov/portal/server.pt/community/healthit_hhs_gov__onc-authorized_testing_and_certification_bodies/3120. Accessed June 28, 2011.
14. Jha AK, DesRoches CM, Campbell EG, et al. Use of electronic health records in U.S. hospitals. N Engl J Med 2009;360(16):1628–38.
15. HIMSS. Stage 7 hospitals. 2010. Available at: http://www.himssanalytics.org/hc_providers/stage7Hospitals.asp. Accessed June 28, 2011.
16. Egger Halbeis CB, Epstein RH, Macario A, et al. Adoption of anesthesia information management systems by academic departments in the United States. Anesth Analg 2008;107(4):1323–9.
17. Sandberg WS. Anesthesia information management systems: almost there. Anesth Analg 2008;107(4):1100–2.

18. Brailer DJ. Guiding the health information technology agenda. Health Aff 2010; 29(4):586–95.
19. Bates DW. The effects of health information technology on inpatient care. Arch Intern Med 2009;169(2):105–7.
20. Amarasingham R, Plantinga L, Diener-West M, et al. Clinical information technologies and inpatient outcomes: a multiple hospital study. Arch Intern Med 2009; 169(2):108–14.
21. Schiff GD, Bates DW. Can electronic clinical documentation help prevent diagnostic errors? N Engl J Med 2010;362(12):1066–9.
22. Gardner RM, Prakash O. Challenges and opportunities for computerizing the anesthesia record. J Clin Anesth 1994;6(4):333–41.
23. Thrush DN. Are automated anesthesia records better? J Clin Anesth 1992;4(5): 386–9.
24. Zollinger RM Jr, Kreul JF, Schneider AJL. Man-made versus computer-generated anesthesia records. J Surg Res 1977;22(4):419–24.
25. Wax DB, Beilin Y, Hossain S, et al. Manual editing of automatically recorded data in an anesthesia information management system. Anesthesiology 2008;109(5): 811–5.
26. Muravchick S, Caldwell JE, Epstein RH, et al. Anesthesia information management system implementation: a practical guide. Anesth Analg 2008;107(5): 1598–608.
27. CMS. Fact sheet: CMS finalizes definition of meaningful use of certified electronic health records (EHR) technology. 2010. Available at: http://www.cms.gov/apps/media/press/factsheet.asp?Counter=3794. Accessed June 28, 2011.
28. Weiner JP, Kfuri T, Chan K, et al. "e-Iatrogenesis": the most critical unintended consequence of CPOE and other HIT. J Am Med Inform Assoc 2007;14(3): 387–8 [discussion: 389].
29. Wachter RM. Expected and unanticipated consequences of the quality and information technology revolutions. JAMA 2006;295(23):2780–3.
30. Hartzband P, Groopman J. Off the record, avoiding the pitfalls of going electronic. N Engl J Med 2008;358(16):1656–8.
31. Compuware. Survey finds healthcare providers unsatisfied with clinical information systems. 2010. Available at: http://www.healthcare-informatics.com/ME2/dirmod.asp?sid=&nm=&type=news&mod=News&mid=9A02E3B96F2A415ABC72CB5F516B4C10&tier=3&nid=32E0CB07AF8D4BE2A6CC2F1FA2429A66. Accessed June 28, 2011.
32. Heeks R. Health information systems: failure, success and improvisation. Int J Med Inform 2006;75(2):125–37.
33. McCarthy C, Eastman D, Garets D. Change management strategies for an effective EMR implementation. Chicago (IL): Healthcare Information and Management Systems Society (HIMSS); 2010.
34. Campbell EM, Sittig DF, Ash JS, et al. Types of unintended consequences related to computerized provider order entry. J Am Med Inform Assoc 2006;13(5):547–56.
35. Ash JS, Sittig DF, Dykstra R, et al. The unintended consequences of computerized provider order entry: findings from a mixed methods exploration. Int J Med Inform 2009;78(Suppl 1):S69–76.
36. Campbell EM, Guappone KP, Sittig DF, et al. Computerized provider order entry adoption: implications for clinical workflow. J Gen Intern Med 2009;24(1):21–6.
37. Saitwal H, Feng X, Walji M, et al. Assessing performance of an Electronic Health Record (EHR) using cognitive task analysis. Int J Med Inform 2010; 79(7):501–6.

38. Koppel R, Metlay JP, Cohen A, et al. Role of computerized physician order entry systems in facilitating medication errors. JAMA 2005;293(10):1197–203.
39. Khajouei R, Jaspers MW. CPOE system design aspects and their qualitative effect on usability. Stud Health Technol Inform 2008;136:309–14.
40. Joint Commission on Accreditation of Healthcare Organizations, USA. Safely implementing health information and converging technologies. Sentinel Event Alert 2008;(42):1–4. Available at: http://www.jointcommission.org/assets/1/18/SEA_42.PDF. Accessed June 28, 2011.
41. Zheng K, Haftel HM, Hirschl RB, et al. Quantifying the impact of health IT implementations on clinical workflow: a new methodological perspective. J Am Med Inform Assoc 2010;17(4):454–61.
42. Koppel R, Wetterneck T, Telles JL, et al. Workarounds to barcode medication administration systems: their occurrences, causes, and threats to patient safety. J Am Med Inform Assoc 2008;15(4):408–23.
43. Armijo D, McDonnell C, Werner K. Electronic health record usability interface design considerations. Rockville (MD): James Bell Assoc for AHRQ, US DHHS; 2009.
44. Beuscart-Zephir MC, Aarts J, Elkin P. Human factors engineering for healthcare IT clinical applications. Int J Med Inform 2010;79(4):223–4.
45. Beuscart-Zephir MC, Pelayo S, Bernonville S. Example of a human factors engineering approach to a medication administration work system: potential impact on patient safety. Int J Med Inform 2010;79(4):e43–57.
46. Hoffman S, Podgurski A. Finding a cure: the case for regulation and oversight of electronic health record systems. Harv J Law Techn 2008;22(1):103–69.
47. Karsh B-T, Weinger MB, Abbott PA, et al. Health information technology: fallacies and sober realities. J Am Med Inform Assoc 2010;17(6):617–23.
48. Sittig DF, Singh H. A new sociotechnical model for studying health information technology in complex adaptive healthcare systems. Qual Saf Health Care 2010;19(Suppl 3):i68–74.
49. Kjeldskov J, Skov MB, Stage J. A longitudinal study of usability in health care: does time heal? Int J Med Inform 2010;79(6):e135–43.
50. Kadry B, Sanderson IC, Macario A. Challenges that limit meaningful use of health information technology. Curr Opin Anaesthesiol 2010;23(2):184–92.
51. Holden RJ. Physicians' beliefs about using EMR and CPOE: in pursuit of a contextualized understanding of health IT use behavior. Int J Med Inform 2010;79(2):71–80.
52. Koppel R, Kreda D. Health care information technology vendors' "Hold Harmless" clause: implications for patients and clinicians. JAMA 2009;301(12):1276–8.
53. Ash JS, Sittig DF, Campbell EM, et al. Some unintended consequences of clinical decision support systems. AMIA Annu Symp Proc 2007;26–30.
54. Ash JS, Sittig DF, Poon EG, et al. The extent and importance of unintended consequences related to computerized provider order entry. J Am Med Inform Assoc 2007;14(4):415–23.
55. Sittig DF, Classen DC. Monitoring and evaluating the use of electronic health records—reply. JAMA 2010;303(19):1918.
56. Koppel R. Monitoring and evaluating the use of electronic health records. JAMA 2010;303(19):1918.
57. Shuren J. Testimony of Jeffrey Shuren, director of FDA's center for devices and radiological health. Washington, DC: Health Information Technology (HIT) Policy Committee, Adoption/Certification Workgroup; 2010.
58. Guerra A. Patient Safety Tops Healthcare Committee's Agenda. Information Week Healthcare. April 22, 2010. Available at: http://www.informationweek.com/news/healthcare/policy/224600030. Accessed June 28, 2011.

59. Thys D. The role of information systems in anesthesia. 2003. Available at: http://www.apsf.org/newsletters/html/2001/summer/03Infosys.htm. Accessed June 28, 2011.

60. Kheterpal S. The intra-operative anesthesia record. APSF Newsletter. 2001. Available at: http://www.apsf.org/newsletters/html/2001/summer/07record.htm. Accessed June 28, 2011.

61. AMA. Medical liability claim frequency: a 2007–2008 snapshot of physicians. Chicago (IL): American Medical Association (AMA); 2010.

62. Kroll DA. The medicolegal aspects of automated anaesthesia records. Clin Anaesthesiol 1990;4(1):237–48.

63. Feldman JM. Medicolegal aspects of anesthesia information management systems. Semin Anesth Perioperat Med Pain 2004;23(2):86–92.

64. Vigoda MM, Lubarsky DA. The medicolegal importance of enhancing timeliness of documentation when using an anesthesia information system and the response to automated feedback in an academic practice. Anesth Analg 2006;103(1):131–6.

65. Hoffman S, Podgurski A. E-Health hazards: provider liability and health record systems. Berkeley Technol Law J 2009;24(4):1524.

66. Dimick C. Shortcuts in electronic records pose risk. J AHIMA 2008;79(6):40–3.

67. World Health Organization (WHO). International Statistical Classification of Diseases and Related Health Problems. New York, NY. Available at: http://www.who.int/classifications/icd/en/. Accessed June 28, 2011.

68. IMO. 60 Revere Drive, Suite 360. Northbrook (IL): Intelligent Medical Objects, Inc; 2010. Available at: http://www.e-imo.com/. Accessed June 28, 2011.

69. APSF. 2010. Available at: http://www.apsf.org/initiatives_data.php. Accessed June 28, 2011.

70. IHTSDO. Snomed-CT. 2010. Available at: http://www.ihtsdo.org/. Accessed June 28, 2011.

71. Saleem JJ, Russ AL, Justice CF, et al. Exploring the persistence of paper with the electronic health record. Int J Med Inform 2009;78(9):618–28.

72. HIMSS. Integration & interoperability. 2010. Available at: http://www.himss.org/ASP/topics_integration.asp. Accessed June 28, 2011.

73. HHS. CONNECT—nationwide health information network. 2010. Available at: http://www.connectopensource.org/about/what-is-CONNECT. Accessed June 28, 2011.

74. Vest JR, Gamm LD. Health information exchange: persistent challenges and new strategies. J Am Med Inform Assoc 2010;17(3):288–94.

75. Delbanco T, Walker J. OpenNotes project. 2010. Available at: http://myopennotes.org/. Accessed June 28, 2011.

76. Reckmann MH, Westbrook JI, Koh Y, et al. Does computerized provider order entry reduce prescribing errors for hospital inpatients? A systematic review. J Am Med Inform Assoc 2009;16(5):613–23.

77. Sittig DF, Wright A, Simonaitis L, et al. The state of the art in clinical knowledge management: an inventory of tools and techniques. Int J Med Inform 2010;79(1):44–57.

78. Kuperman GJ, Bobb A, Payne TH, et al. Medication-related clinical decision support in computerized provider order entry systems: a review. J Am Med Inform Assoc 2007;14(1):29–40.

79. Shojania KG, Jennings A, Mayhew A, et al. Effect of point-of-care computer reminders on physician behaviour: a systematic review. CMAJ 2010;182(5):E216–25.

80. Leapfrog. Leapfrog group report on CPOE evaluation tool results, June 2008 to January 2010. Washington, DC: The Leapfrog Group; 2010. Available at: http://www.leapfroggroup.org/media/file/NewCPOEEvaluationToolResultsReport.pdf. Accessed June 28, 2011.

81. Sandberg WS, Sandberg EH, Seim AR, et al. Real-time checking of electronic anesthesia records for documentation errors and automatically text messaging clinicians improves quality of documentation. Anesth Analg 2008;106(1): 192–201.
82. Epstein RH. Postoperative nausea and vomiting, decision support, and regulatory oversight. Anesth Analg 2010;111(2):270–1.
83. Epstein RH, Dexter F, Piotrowski E. Automated correction of room location errors in anesthesia information management systems. Anesth Analg 2008;107(3): 965–71.

SECTION 2:
Computers in Anesthesia

Advanced Integrated Real-Time Clinical Displays

Grant H. Kruger, PhD[a,b,]*, Kevin K. Tremper, MD, PhD[a]

KEYWORDS

- Patient monitoring • Clinical display • Patient safety
- Decision support

Even though anesthesiology has been a leader in patient safety efforts and has dramatically improved mortality rates, errors still occur, resulting in patient mortality or morbidity.[1–5] Additionally, modern research tools and techniques have allowed the influence of preoperative patient data on intraoperative anesthesia provision and, subsequently, on postoperative patient outcomes to be studied. This information is resulting in the emergence of far more complex treatment scenarios, with multitudes of specific treatment regimes that need to be memorized and instantly recalled by physicians to optimize patient outcomes.

Information overload of the anesthesiologist and other acute care practitioners from existing and additional demands through technological advances may threaten the safety of patients in the intensive care unit (ICU) or under anesthesia in the operating room (OR). This circumstance has mainly been driven by the increase in the number and complexity of equipment used to control and monitor the vital functions of patients over the years. Modern anesthesia monitors are able to provide more than 20 periodic or continuous traces regarding the status of patients.[6] The number and complexity of devices and alarms monitoring patient physiologic parameters fight for the anesthesiologist's attention as the human brain can only assimilate, integrate, and act on a certain amount of information at one time.[6–8]

This article focuses on discussing aspects of human-in-the-loop control methodology as applied to the medical domain, followed by the limitations and problems this approach presents. The authors briefly discuss electronic medical records as

Support was provided solely from institutional or departmental sources.

The University of Michigan has filed software patents regarding display technology described in this article.

[a] Department of Anesthesiology, University of Michigan Medical School, 1500 East Medical Center Drive, Ann Arbor, MI 48109-5048, USA

[b] Department of Mechanical Engineering, University of Michigan, 2350 Hayward Street, Ann Arbor, MI 48109, USA

* Corresponding author. Department of Mechanical Engineering, University of Michigan, 2350 Hayward Street, Ann Arbor, MI 48109.

E-mail address: ghkruger@med.umich.edu

Anesthesiology Clin 29 (2011) 487–504

doi:10.1016/j.anclin.2011.05.004

1932-2275/11/$ – see front matter © 2011 Elsevier Inc. All rights reserved.

the current state of the art that hospitals are adopting for patient monitoring and their untapped potential for empowering advanced displays to realize next-generation patient care. Next the authors propose artificial intelligence as an enabling technology to drive the smart displays of the future, using intelligent software agent-based decision-support technology that operates alongside physicians to overcome the limitations of human-in-the-loop control. The article concludes by presenting a system developed by the University of Michigan to address the future of intelligent patient care.

PATIENT MONITORING AND HUMAN-IN-THE-LOOP CONTROL

In many fields, standard displays merely provide the convenient reproduction of a measured quantity to allow operators to observe the operation of a system. Of course this makes the assumption that the quantities measured and displayed adequately describe the system state. The task of assimilating and integrating these quantities in both space and time is the responsibility of the operator. Optionally, thresholds can be applied to the monitored quantities and generate alerts, either audio, visual, or some combination of both, so that the operator can take action if the quantity is out of the acceptable range and this is missed by the operator. At this point it should be noted that this is the most basic form of advanced intelligent display: the system being monitored is able to detect a deviation from the accepted normal operation, as monitored through some quantity, and then effect an action (via the operator) to make a change to correct the situation. This human-in-the-loop type of process monitoring and control is illustrated in **Fig. 1**. The display is only the visible component of a much more complex system running in the background, which forms the advanced portion of the display. A good analogy would be that of an iceberg, where only a small fraction is visible above the surface of the water. Because many systems are very complex (ie, the human body under anesthesia), they require humans in the control loop to refine or validate the final control decision and effect the change to ensure a safe return to normal operation.

Patients in the OR and ICU are surrounded by a multitude of medical devices (vital sign monitors, therapeutic devices supporting/replacing organs, fluid, gas or medication administration devices).[7] In these environments, patient monitoring can be performed with any combination of continuous, periodic, or alert-driven intervals.[1] For this discussion, monitoring is defined as an intentional action by the physician to observe some aspect regarding the state of patients. At first glance, continuous monitoring (usually in the OR) may seem like a reliable situation; however, procedural and clinical limitations make this complicated to achieve in reality and may result in information overload for clinicians.

Anesthesiologists have to continually switch between screens to scan historic time series trends for relative changes and to look at multiple devices for additional information to detect patient deterioration and make diagnoses, which usually requires some urgency.[7,8] Because human concentration decreases as a function of time and intensity (amount of incoming information), it can be very difficult to maintain

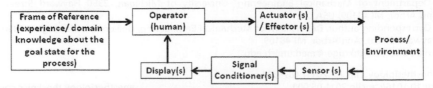

Fig. 1. Human-in-the-loop monitoring and control.

perfect vigilance through a lengthy case.[7] The constant level of vigilance necessary while monitoring variables and alarm management can take its toll on the anesthesiologist, rapidly degrading the quality of human-based monitoring.[7] Additionally, slow-to-develop conditions can be difficult to detect because of the nonperiodic nature of this method.[6] Continuous monitoring quickly deteriorates as the monitored system becomes more complex and a greater number of quantities need to be monitored to fully observe the system.

Periodic monitoring according to a schedule is the only practical way clinicians can monitor groups of patients in the ICU, or multiple real-time physiologic measurements from a single patient in the OR. Because of the nature of this monitoring modality it is inevitable that events will be missed, potentially harming patients or affecting outcomes.

This situation motivates the use of alert-driven monitoring to attract the physician's attention if a signal falls outside a specified range.[6] Physiologic signals from patients are continuously recorded and clinicians are only informed when abnormalities are detected. Alert driven monitoring presents a method that can be used in conjunction with continuous and periodic monitoring to improve both these methods and potentially overcome some of the limitations of human-in-the-loop control.

Practically, however, instead of providing the additional diagnosis benefit, most physiologic variable traces or alerts are frequently turned off to prevent distraction caused by confusing or false alarms resulting in information overload.[6–9] A survey conducted by McIntyre[10] found that 58% of the 789 anesthesiologists questioned admitted to muting an alarm for a variety of reasons. An alternative to turning off alarms is setting safe limits to reduce the frequency of false alarms; however, this can result in the unnecessary deterioration of a patient's condition in the event of a true alarm.[7,9] Even though alert-driven monitoring is an improvement to other methods, the situation is still fraught with many challenges.

THE CHALLENGES OF ALERT-DRIVEN MONITORING

In the OR and ICU, multitudes of false alarms frequently occur, whereas only a few may provide useful information to the anesthesiologist. This high false-positive rate potentially leads to the desensitization toward true alarms.[8,9,11] Research by Imhoff and colleagues[9] reported that approximately 90% of all alarms in critical-care monitoring are false positives. In a study by Chambrin and colleagues,[12] no medical action was taken for 72% of all the alarms. The positive predictive value was only 27% and the specificity was only 58%. The negative predictive value and the sensitivity were 99% and 97%, respectively.

Additionally, if several audio alerts fire simultaneously, similar tones or more intense tones can mask other alerts and it can waste valuable time and increase anxiety for the anesthesiologist to rank the various alerts by severity and locate the source of the alarm, especially because certain alarms (eg, hypotension) can have multiple causes. Standards for alarms between manufactures are limited or nonexistent, which can result in different alerts from equipment that performs the same function. There is also little relationship between medical situation urgency and the type of alarm; for example, a feeding pump may produce a more critical-sounding alert than a ventilator alarm, which can be misleading. This circumstance further leads to situations where certain alarms can mask other alarms because of their acoustic similarity or intensity.[8] Research has shown that critical care nurses can only identify a few of the many alert sounds correctly.[8,9] A study in a Canadian hospital by Momtahan and Tansley[13] revealed that only 39% of ICU nurses and 40% of anesthesiologists could correctly identify audio warnings.

A typical cardiothoracic OR can have about 18 different alarms providing a mix of visual and audio alerts.[7] Meijler[14] analyzed 731 warnings generated by a statistical disturbance algorithm during cardiac surgery by linking them to the response of the anesthesiologist. Of these alerts, 7% were useful, and 13% followed some intervention and probably could have been predicted and eliminated. Kestin and colleagues[15] evaluated the significance of auditory alarms during the routine anesthetic management of 50 pediatric patients undergoing elective surgery. Five monitors with auditory alarms were used routinely: electrocardiogram (ECG), automatic blood pressure, oxygen analyzer, pulse oximeter, and ventilator low pressure (disconnect alarm). There was a mean of 10 alarms per case, with an average frequency of 1 alarm every 4.5 minutes. The incidence of alarms varied little between the different phases of anesthesia and surgery. Of all alarms that sounded, 75 % were spurious (eg, caused by patient movement, interference, or mechanical problems). Only 3% of all alarms indicated risk to the patient. O'Carroll[16] recorded a total of 1455 alarms during a 3-week period. Only 8 indicated a potentially serious threat to patient safety: 1 ventilator disconnect alarm and 7 dysrhythmias. Lawless[17] found that the rate of true alarms in the pediatric ICU was about 10%; various procedures induced 27% of the alarms and 68% were truly false alarms. In another study, approximately one-third of all alarms originated from the ventilator, another third from the cardiovascular monitor, and 15% from pulse oximetry. Similar studies found pulse oximetry to cause more than 40% of all false alarms. In patients with invasive blood-pressure monitoring, arterial blood-pressure alarms can also often be the leading cause of false alarms.[9]

These situations could be attributed to the poor interoperability between medical devices and the current lack of standardization of alerts and communication protocols. The current lack of integration between medical devices and displays results in each system having their own specialized threshold-based visual or acoustic alarms relating to some aspect of the state of patients or equipment.[7,9,18] Because there is little redundancy in the signals against which to validate the physiologic state of patients, some care-related activity (sensor movement, accidental disconnections, and so forth) may result in a series of false alarms, reducing the specificity of the alerts.[6,7,9] In a research study by Imhoff and colleagues,[19] 40% of all alarms resulted from patient manipulation. This situation, coupled with the various common surgical distractions and tasks the anesthesiologist must perform, can still make it easy to miss physiologic variable changes or diagnoses relying on historic sensor data (eg, potential hypotension). These factors, along with the associated anxiety, limit the time available to observe and treat the cause of alarms.[6-8]

If not well managed, alert-driven monitoring may not provide the promised solution and may even distract clinicians. It can clearly be seen that alarms are necessary, but not in large numbers. A reduction in the unacceptably high incidence of false or spurious alarms during routine anesthesia monitoring would contribute to the proper use of alarms.[7] One potential solution to this problem is through the use of integrated monitoring and displays, using redundant information from multiple sources to automatically validate alerts.

ELECTRONIC MEDICAL RECORDS FOR INTEGRATED PATIENT MONITORING

The process of integrating the various sources of medical data has already begun through the collection of data into a variety of databases and computerized records in the form of the electronic medical record (EMR). This process is already commonplace at many hospitals through sensors attached to patients (such as in the OR or ICU), automated laboratory equipment, and manual entry by clinicians. The vision presented in an article by Dear and colleagues[20] in 1999 for an EMR where all information is electronically entered (via keyboard, touch screen, or voice control) and seamlessly added to the record has been mostly achieved.

However, even though the EMR is replacing its paper-based counterpart, the opportunity to change workflow and the overall process of care has not yet been fully realized.[21] It is clear that simply viewing and recording information, as is currently the case with EMRs, is not sufficient to realize improved quality of patient care. The data contained in EMRs, including past and real-time physiologic data, should be continuously synthesized to extract critical information describing the overall state of patients and the care necessary.[20] This information can improve alarm accuracy for the prediction of impending dangerous situations for patients, such as drug interactions, postoperative morbidity, and so forth.[6] This point is especially true as the complexity of modern anesthesiology and surgery increases, which requires an increased awareness from anesthesiologists to maintain patient safety and improve outcomes.[7]

EMRs provide the foundation for the next generation of integrated monitoring, display, alert, and decision support systems (DSS), where signals from all physiologic monitors are analyzed by a centralized processing facility. In these next-generation systems, it can be hypothesized that anesthesiologists would have all relevant medical information concerning patients, including high sensitivity and specificity alarm conditions, potential risk factors, and suggestions for care provision (based on published medical theory), presented on a single computer screen.[7] There would be no need to scan for information from several pieces of equipment because data from a variety of monitors can be combined using mathematical modeling and rule-based logic into meaningful quantitative statements about the functioning of specific organ systems.

It is thought that integrated intelligent monitoring systems are able to detect deviations and states that may not be noticed or recognized through periodic clinical observations alone and prevent adverse patient outcomes.[7] The current fundamental challenge of intelligent patient-monitoring systems is how to integrate them with conventional systems in a way that reduces processing load on the anesthesiologist while not negatively impacting patient care.[6]

CHALLENGES FACING SMART DISPLAYS

As EMR databases grow, powerful methods are necessary to convert this data into information. Classical computing methods are not sufficient when attempting to model complex medical problems with a variety of user and parameter interactions.[19] Additionally, new advanced display and alarm methods will need to fulfill several methodological criteria, such as good systems practices (eg, robustness), software (eg, extensibility), and regulatory and patient care practices (eg, applicability to large patient populations). Similar technology is starting to become available for limited domains, such as for intelligent ECG analysis and pulmonary function measurement.[22] However, there is much more progress that needs to be made before these systems will be suitable for wide-scale use in general anesthesia cases.

An immediate and very practical challenge of the integrated advanced monitoring approach demands the full integration of monitoring equipment in the OR, ICU, laboratories, medical records and the availability to appropriate protocols to access these resources.[7] Currently, data from these sources are not in a single database or easily usable format.[23] Groups have developed, and are still developing, globally applicable medical device communication standards, such as Digital Imaging and Communications in Medicine (imaging), Health Level-7 (messaging), Institute of Electrical and Electronics Engineers/International Organization for Standardization 11073, and

CANopen, to name a few. However, not all protocols provide the necessary functionality for all medical applications, and medical device manufacturers seem to prefer their own propriety solutions.

Other methodological aspects to consider are how this continually growing medical knowledge base should be represented in a comprehensive, extensible, and usable fashion. The time course over which various data are acquired varies significantly from seconds to hours, as does its representation (encoding format) in the system. This variation means that the validity of the confidence associated with a measurement may vary over time or as the patients treatment regime is varied, which further complicates inferences based on this data.

A more fundamental challenge to overcome in medical domains is that no detailed comprehensive models exist for human physiologic processes, behaviors, and interactions, other than some isolated fragments of knowledge.[24] Physicians and nurses are motivated to make decisions based on the available data as well as their internal cognitive models of the system. These models may be based on accepted best practices, past experience, and intuition. For DSSs, to provide similar insight as clinicians requires comprehensive models of important aspects of human physiologic and disease processes. Univariate and multivariate methods have been proposed and investigated, mostly from the fields of statistics and artificial intelligence (AI). Some have even shown encouraging results in clinical studies.[9]

AI is currently included as part of accepted software technology solutions in certain fields, such as logistics, data mining, and image processing. Generally, AI proposes methodologies and algorithms that are able to provide solutions to problems similar to those a specialist in that domain would provide if presented with the same problem. AI has boosted discovery in genetics and molecular medicine by providing machine learning algorithms, knowledge representation, biomedical ontologies, and natural language processing tools.[24] Traditionally, AI systems consisted of a singular algorithm (eg, Expert Systems, Neural Network, Fuzzy Logic, and so forth) with an associated methodology of how the algorithms would be integrated with the target system. Single algorithm standalone AI systems usually only provide acceptable solutions over limited problem domains and cannot deal with overly complex problems. These forms of AI have been widely used in medical DSSs; however, few have been widely accepted into clinical practice.[25–27] A well-known clinical DSS is Mycin, which is a consultation system that used simple pattern matching for the diagnosis and therapy selection of patients with bacterial infections.[28] The Internist-1 expert system modeled clinicians' behavior to diagnose multiple diseases and performed favorably in certain areas of the internal medical domain.[29] A clinical DDS based on Causal Associational Networks (CASNET), for general computer-assisted medical decision making has been previously investigated for the diagnosis and treatment of glaucoma.[30] In 2008, Wadhwa[26] presented an analysis of a failed clinical rule-based DSS for congestive heart failure. However, an excessive number of alerts for chronic heart failure occurred for the majority of patients. Another study in 2008 by Toth-Pal[27] used an Internet-based application for the management of chronic heart failure to determine the general practitioner attitudes and acceptance of DSS systems. Stevenson and colleagues[25] studied the implementation of DSSs to rural hospitals using an Internet-based clinical DSS designed to optimize antimicrobial prescriptions for pneumonia in 5 rural hospitals. Key findings of this and other investigations into why these systems did not fully meet the clinical needs included organizational and cultural barriers, such as ease of use; consistent reliable advice; and seamless integration with existing workflow. Barriers to acceptance have were insufficient level of computer skills and time constraints.[27] An emerging trend in DSSs is that false alarms are prevalent (up to 90% in some cases) and, thus, easily ignored. Many DSSs do not integrate into existing electronic systems or even usual practices of care, and the effects on patient outcomes are inconclusive.[12,17,31–35]

AI medical research has moved away from standalone AI systems, and systems integrated with medical data warehouses are growing in popularity for addressing the shortcomings of standalone AI. These systems integrate EMR, order entry, and laboratory systems with a wide variety of computational methods.[24] Software agent technology is emerging as one of the new promising paradigms focused on modeling, design, and development of complex intelligent systems with the hope of improving the performance of DSSs.[36]

INTELLIGENT AGENTS FOR ADVANCED SMART DISPLAYS

An agent can be defined as a software entity (object) operating with a certain degree of autonomy in a particular environment to accomplish the goals prescribed by its end user according to a certain defined behavior, possibly with the aid of other agents. Agents offer benefits over traditional software approaches as far as reusability, reliability, flexibility, robustness, maintainability, and adaptability are concerned. Agent technology supports integration of legacy systems and overcomes problems of centralized systems. These problems include performance bottlenecks, resource limitations, and various failure modes.[36] Adaptive and intelligent agents (IA) are able to pursue multiple goals in dynamic, complex, and uncertain environments, such as the critical care environment, and are already being applied to areas of the medical field, including medical data management, planning and resource allocation, decision support systems, remote care/telemedicine/pervasive care, and hybrid approaches. Generally, agent-based systems consist of a group of independent entities that each have specialized functions, such as planning, monitoring, searching, and so forth, and communicate via well-defined interfaces. Each entity and agent system as a whole performs 3 functions: (1) perception of its physical environment, (2) effect changes to the environment, and (3) action computation to decide on the change necessary to move closer to a goal (improved patient outcomes/safety) as defined by a performance measure. Entities will request assistance from other, more specialized entities to complete a complex task. Some critical characteristics of an IA are autonomy, reactivity (to change in environment), and rationality (make correct decisions a professional would make given the same data). There are 3 major foci that must be investigated to develop robust systems that seamlessly integrate with clinical practice: medical information system integration, complex systems modeling using uncertain knowledge, and clinical interfacing. Most modern medical DSSs use a user agent (advanced display), often Internet based, to allow clinicians to present a problem that needs to be solved and analyze the proposed solution.[36] Examples of medical data management system agents that collect (possibly from distributed sources), filter, and organize this information include the national electronic library for health, virtual electronic patient record, or context-aware hospital information system. Planning and resource allocation agents that make scheduling and planning decisions for hospital workflow examples include Protégé, Agent.Hospital, Carrel (Barcelona), or the Medical Information Agent (Amsterdam). Singh and colleagues[37,38] presented an agent-based health care intelligent assistant designed for clinicians to retrieve and use geographically distributed organizational knowledge to solve medical episodes. The system used case-based reasoning to use encoded knowledge from past cases to classify new cases. The system used a star-based topology with 2 central agents (manager agent and master presentation agent), a web server agent for user interaction, with each case having a case-broker agent and presentation agent pair.[36] The HealthAgents system developed by Gonzalez-Velez and colleagues[39] integrated novel pattern-recognition discrimination methods to analyze magnetic resonance imaging and DNA micro-array data. The system uses networked agents able to access a global knowledge repository consisting of multiple medical centers for brain tumor diagnosis and prognosis. Each node consists of a classifier and graphical user interface (GUI) agent able to communicate with local devices (database, classifier, physicians, and so forth). The directory facilitator agent allows searches of all nodes. Clinicians can access the system via the GUI agents. Each node consists of its own set of cases and machine learning algorithms. The results returned from the nodes reflect diagnosis from different points of view. Health Care Services (HeCaSe2) is another distributed autonomous agent platform to deliver health care services to clinicians and patients. The system consists of a user agent that interacts with patients and stores their static and dynamic data. A broker agent keeps track of all the medical centers in an area, whereas the medical center agent manages the accesses to agents within a medical center. Each department is represented by a department agent, containing a set of services. These services are delivered by agents linked to human or physical resources through appropriate interfaces. In addition to the service agent, there is a doctor, guideline, ontology, and medical record agent. Aingeru (Interoperable Databases Group, Basque, Spain) is an agent-based pervasive care system using PDAs for continuous monitoring of elderly persons via PDA-based sensors using sensor agents.[36] The PDA analyzes the data using the conditions checker (reasoning) agent locally, and only alerts are transmitted via the cellular network based General Packet Radio Service (GPRS). Koutkias and colleagues,[40] developed a rule-based pervasive care system to enhance monitoring, surveillance and educational services for the management of chronic diseases. The system is located in departments that mediate between clinicians and patients seeking advice or therapy. The system monitors the current status from sensors to proactively detect anomalous cases and alerts clinicians. Cervantes and colleagues[41] present a pervasive care system using multiple agents and neural networks to form a DSS for the management of chronic patients. Physiologic data are sequentially collected by dynamically reconfigurable sensor agents and evaluated by the patient agent to detect emergent symptoms (using, for example, utility-based methods, rule-based approaches, and analysis of time series) and the current state of the patient (using, for example, neural network-based pattern recognition). A mobile doctor agent manages the transport of medical data.

Researchers at the University of Michigan (UM) have developed a basic general-purpose IA architecture capable of integrating the data from various sources, such as EMRs, patient monitors, anesthesia machines, and so forth, in the ICU and OR.[42] This system is briefly discussed in the following section.

THE RISKWATCH INTEGRATED ADVANCED SMART DISPLAY SYSTEM

A UM IA system is being developed to provide graphical summaries and alerts based on the physiologic state of patients. It is able to perform basic decision support by implementing expert rules captured from anesthesiologists and critical care clinicians. The system supports multiple agents, each consisting of an input, processing, and output method. In the medical domain, it is extremely important that an intelligent system make rational decisions. A medical rational decision can be defined as a decision that mimics that of an experienced physician if given the same facts. **Fig. 2** illustrates this

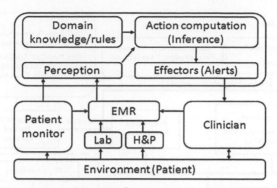

Fig. 2. Reactive agent system architecture for patient supervision. H&P, history and physical.

conceptual architecture of this agent system. Three key agents (perception, action computation and effector agents) work together to achieve rational behavior.

The perception agent is responsible for capturing data describing the environment (the patient) by capturing information from patient monitors and integrating the data from the history and physical (H&P) EMR. The ability of the agent to perceive its environment is essential to enable the agent to make rational decisions. Key steps for accurate perception include the sensor selection, data cleaning, and data integration from various heterogeneous data sources (ie, EMRs, patient monitors, anesthesia information systems, clinicians).

The action computation agent analyzes the perceived data and determines the state of the patient. The patient state is predicted based on knowledge about human physiology, encoded as a combination of mathematical models and production rules. The agent then decides what it needs to convey to the clinician to effect the required change in the physiologic state of the patient. This communication could be as simple as displaying flashing text and playing an audio alert.

Finally, an effector agent interfaces with clinicians through a GUI and an audio alert system. The primary goal for this agent is to convey the current physiologic state of patients in a clear and concise format as well as inform the clinician to any abnormal conditions.

Using this architecture, the authors are able to perform various types of intelligent signal processing, visualization, and alerting to implement and study the performance of artifact removal, classification/diagnosis, decision support, and prediction algorithms. There is no need for clinicians to scan for information from several pieces of equipment because data from a variety of monitors are combined using mathematical modeling and rule-based logic into meaningful statements about the patient state. The system is designed to provide supervisory support to the caregiver and not interfere or replace existing workflow policies. A key aspect of agents is their communication ability, allowing them to share information with other agents and distributed hospital systems. Even though this is a simple agent system for this environment, it can be seen that many specialized agents (ie, to predict the occurrence of special conditions/diseases) could be developed, which function together to improve multiple aspects of patient care.

PERCEPTION AGENT

Fig. 3 illustrates the physical implementation and network infrastructure of the agent system on the UM Medical Center's 14-bed cardiothoracic ICU. This area uses Solar

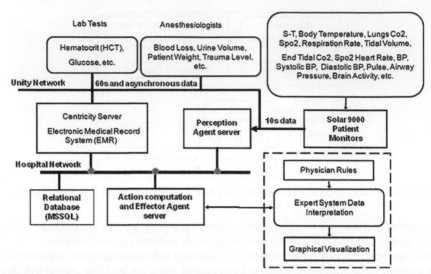

Fig. 3. Network architecture of the Riskwatch system. BP, blood pressure; MSSQL, Microsoft Structured Query Language. (*Courtesy of* the University of Michigan, Ann Arbor, Michigan; with permission.)

9000 monitors (General Electric Healthcare WI, USA), which pass data to a common data network (Unity Network, General Electric Healthcare), similar to other monitor systems. A software package (Monitor Capture Server, General Electric Healthcare) was used to capture the physiologic data broadcast over the network by the monitors. This package then logs the data to a SQL database (SQL Server, Microsoft Corporation, Redmond, WA, USA) in a standard format every 10 seconds. The UM hospital uses the Centricity EMR (General Electric Healthcare) to capture and store patient records (H&P), OR scheduling, anesthesia records, and so forth. The anesthesia record contains key surgical events (anesthesia start, incision, and so forth), lab values, fluid balance (ins and outs), drugs, and physiologic data from the patient monitor. A multi-threaded Java based server integrates real-time patient monitor data using a SQL query through the Java Database Connectivity (JDBC) connector every 2 seconds. Another query is performed on the EMR using stored procedures every minute. The patient monitor data and EMR data are integrated and cleaned. Certain surgeries use different sets of sensors, with multiple sensors measuring similar quantities (eg, pulse oximeter heart rate and ECG heart rate, or systolic pressure variation, central venous pressure, and pulmonary artery pressure). In these situations, the sensor providing the cleaner signal is automatically chosen. When the action computation agent connects to the perception agent, it opens a transmission control protocol (TCP) socket for mutual communication and the optimal set of data describing the patient state is continually updated.

ACTION COMPUTATION AGENT

Production rules are created for alerts, notifications, and reminders. Alerts are combinations of 1 or several monitors, EMR, or calculated variables that may potentially cause adverse outcomes if not addressed in a timely manner. An example of

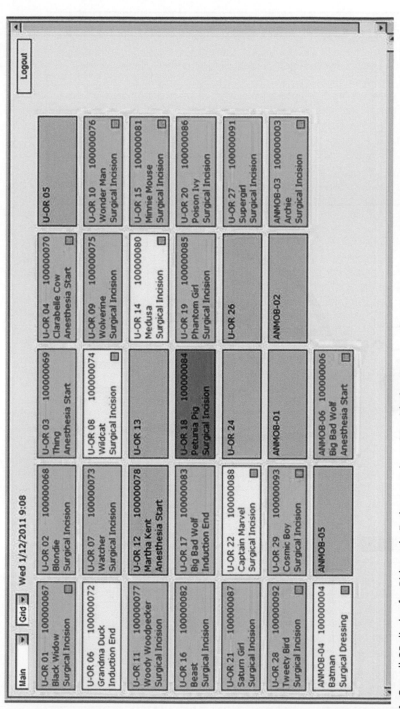

Fig. 4. Overall OR display for Riskwatch. Each square is an OR with the room number, patient name, and status of the case (eg, surgical incision, anesthesia start, surgical dressing). The color green designates that all monitored systems are in the normal range; the color yellow designates that at least 1 system is in a marginal range; and the color red designates that at least 1 system is in an abnormal range. The small orange squares inside the boxes designate that at least 1 system has risk factors. (*Courtesy of* the University of Michigan, Ann Arbor, Michigan; with permission.)

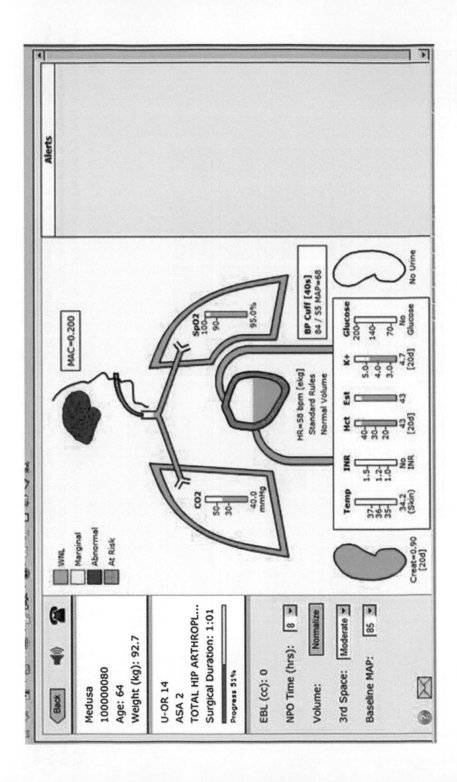

a production rule used by the system to detect long-term hypotension in the ICU is presented as Equation 1. In this specific implementation, all the consequent terms were the same, resulting in an alarm being generated, and a unity certainty value was assumed for all rules. For the rules that follow, Δt, represents the difference in time between the first occurrence of the first term of the antecedent and the time the current inference is occurring. The bar above the physiologic variables indicates that they have been passed through the median filter. Of course, a significantly more complex hierarchy of production rules could be used, including vectors for rule certainty and support; however, for the authors' preliminary analysis, it was thought that a more fundamental study should initially be performed that can be more readily related to the current situation in the ICU.

$$P1 : (\overline{SBP}<80 \text{ mm Hg}) \wedge (\Delta t>30 \text{ min}) \rightarrow alarm\_SBP30 \tag{1}$$

$$h(t) = h_0/e^{b(t)/V} \tag{2}$$

$$P4 : (\overline{SBP}<60) \wedge (PAP>50) \wedge (PEEP>20) \rightarrow alarm4 \tag{3}$$

For the OR agent system, notification rules contain normal, abnormal, and marginal ranges for variables, such as bispectral index, systolic blood pressure (SBP), heart filling volume (based on a continuous input and output time-based calculation and fluids entered in the EMR), end tidal (ET) CO_2, peak airway pressure (PAP), positive end-expiratory pressure (PEEP), pulse oximeter oxygen saturation (SpO_2), body temperature, hematocrit (HCT), estimated HCT, glucose, and creatine. All the rules and thresholds are based on well-defined and agreed upon anesthesia practice. Equation 2 provides an example of an equation used to predict a patient's estimated HCT during surgery,[43] where, $b(t)$ is the estimated blood loss, taking into account any transfusions; h_0 is the last hematocrit measurement; and $h(t)$ corresponds to the estimated hematocrit at time interval t. V is the estimated body volume calculated by multiplying the body weight by 70 mL. Equation 3 presents an example of an OR-type alert rule that detects probable tension pneumothorax (alarm 4). Reminders alert the physician to provide some treatment, remind them to perform certain duties, or highlight the current patient states.

Fig. 5. A Riskwatch display of 1 patient, the icons for each organ are self-evident, the lungs ventilate up and down with respiration, and the heart beats with heart rate. The left side of the screen shows case information, including current progress of case and percent completion, EBL, NPO hours, and preoperative baseline mean arterial pressure. The color code: green is normal, yellow is marginal, red is abnormal, and orange demonstrates organ system at risk. In this case, part of the patient's brain is orange, which indicates that he or she has a history of stroke; and the heart is orange, designating a cardiac history. This figure shows the heart volume to be low, which is based on an input/output (IO) calculation unless there is an objective measure, such as systolic pressure variation (SPV) or CVP or PAW. In this figure, an SPV of 11 demonstrates the heart filling volume is a bit low. The square at the bottom between the kidneys shows the current laboratory values and the last time they were drawn. This case shows a glucose of 222, which is a high value and is colored red, and was drawn 32 minutes ago. There is also an alert portion of the screen on the right; in this case, it recommends starting an insulin infusion of 1 unit per hour. BP, blood pressure; CVP, central venous pressure; EBL, estimated blood loss; MAP, mean arterial pressure; NPO, nil per os; PAW, pulmonary artery wedge pressure. (*Courtesy of* the University of Michigan, Ann Arbor, Michigan; with permission.)

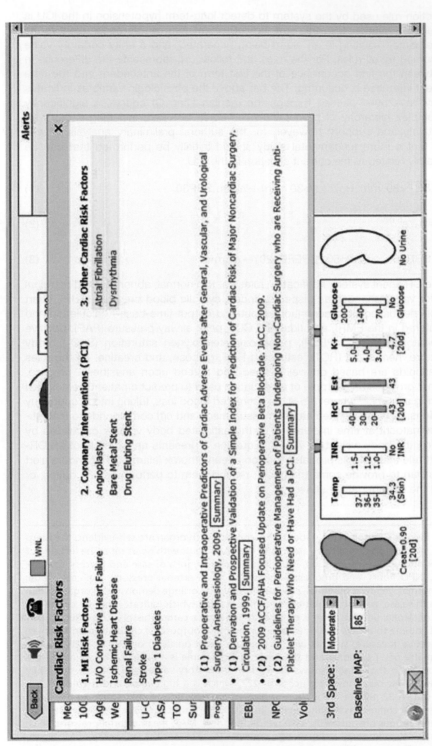

Fig. 6. If any organ at risk is selected (the screen is touched), a window will open; in this case it is the heart. On the left, the MI risk factors are listed; the history of coronary intervention is in the middle; and a list of other cardiac problems is on the right. If the patient has these risk factors, they are highlighted in yellow. Below this are pertinent references and guidelines for cardiac care. In this case, the patient has a history of atrial fibrillation. H/O, history of; MI, myocardial infarction; PCI, percutaneous coronary intervention. (*Courtesy of* the University of Michigan, Ann Arbor, Michigan; with permission.)

EFFECTOR METHOD (ADVANCED DISPLAY AND ALERTS)

The patient-state visualization system was developed using Internet-based techniques (Adobe Flex; Adobe Systems Incorporated, USA). The interface integrates and displays the patient state, critical variables, and presents alerts and alarms as dictated by the action computation agent. The system logs all alerts and alarms fired in an SQL database for retrospective analysis. **Fig. 4** provides a screen shot of the GUI, providing a high-level overview of a set of ORs at UM. Each square designates an OR and the color signifies an alert status: green demonstrates all monitored parameters in the normal range, yellow demonstrates some of the monitored parameters that are in the margin range, and red demonstrates that some are in the abnormal range. The small orange squares signify that the patient has comorbidities for one of the monitored organ systems. **Fig. 5** is a display of an individual patient where the heart is beating, live, in time with the EKG heart rate, and the lungs are inflating with the respiratory rate. On the upper left of the figure is a color-coded key designating normal, marginal, abnormal, and system at risk. The left side of the figure designates case details and the right side will signify alerts. Laboratory values and the temperature are in the square at the bottom of the figure, between the two kidneys. There is continuous monitoring of monitored anesthesia care (MAC), ventilation, oxygenation, blood pressure, and estimated filling volume. The volume of the heart goes up and down with a continuous input/output (IO) calculation for the patients' fluid status. The trachea color indicates the PAP, and the color of the lung's border indicates the PEEP. A gauge inside the left lung indicates the $ETCO_2$ and the right lung shows SpO_2. Similar graphical color-coded alerts apply to the other areas. **Fig. 6** is the display that opens when an organ is at risk; in this case, the heart is selected (the screen is touched). The left of the figure shows the presence of coronary interventions and on the right it lists other coronary risk factors. Below these are the selected references and guidelines. For the OR-based agent system, all real-time variables displayed contain the corresponding measured value and time difference between the last update and current time (dt). If dt is too large, then the values displayed will be replaced with a message indicating the variable is no longer available (ie, no blood pressure [BP]). If an alert is fired, an intuitive message will appear together with the alarm tone to draw the attention of the physician. The reset button acknowledges all alarms that are currently activated. When an alarm is active, an alert tone is sounded once to attract the physician's attention. The physician can silence or resume the alarm by pressing the silence button. If the cause of the alarm is not addressed, the alarming tone will repeat automatically in 1 minute.

SUMMARY

Information overload of the anesthesiologist and other acute care practitioners from existing and additional demands caused by technological advances and distractions related to patient care provision may negatively impact outcomes and the safety of patients under anesthesia in the OR and ICU. This information overload is mainly caused by shortcomings of human-in-the-loop monitoring and control and the poor specificity of physiologic alarms. Even though dozens of traditional computer-based DSSs have been developed and tested, few have been widely accepted into clinical practice. The last 2 decades have seen many researchers study clinical alerting algorithms and displays, but there has been little progress in the development and implementation of smart alarms and monitoring systems exhibiting high sensitivity and specificity in routine practice. The new introduction of EMRs has facilitated the integration of patient information from multiple sources. However, comparatively little has been done as of yet to harness the full potential of the data integration offered by EMRs to provide additional information in real time at the point of care and to generate high sensitivity and specificity alerts. Modern AI techniques, such as IAs, have shown great potential in various domains and they appear to be able to meet the need of more intelligent displays for improving patient outcomes in the future.

The integration of EMRs, clinical DSSs, and multi-agent systems in real health care settings still has a long way to go to achieve their desired goals. However, preliminary results are promising, making intelligent DSS based patient monitoring a fertile area for cutting-edge research to improve patient outcomes. There are 3 key research focus areas: (1) methods for the design of these systems for the seamless integration into clinical practice and bridge the gap between academic prototypes, (2) how to represent and integrate various types of medical domain knowledge into comprehensive physiologic and disease models, and (3) advanced algorithms to use this domain knowledge for high sensitivity and specificity alerts. It is clear that as technology advances, displays will become more intelligent. There are many ways to achieve this; however, generally this requires improved monitoring of the observed environment, through additional sensors or sensor integration and more advanced algorithms to model or classify signals, so that higher-level alerts with higher positive predictive characteristics and specificities can be realized. Next-generation DSSs are set to improve patient outcomes in the future by incorporating advanced AI methods, such as IAs, based on top of EMRs systems and incorporating novel visual and acoustic alert systems.

REFERENCES

1. Sneha S, Varshney U. Enabling ubiquitous monitoring: model, decision protocols, opportunities and challenges. Decis Support Syst 2009;46:606–19.
2. Committee on Quality of Health Care in America, Institute of Medicine. In: Kohn LT, Corrigan JM, Donaldson MS, editors. To err is human: building a safer health system. Washington, DC: National Academy Press; 2000. p. 287.
3. Botney R. Improving patient safety in anesthesia: a success story? Int J Radiat Oncol Biol Phys 2008;71(1):S182–6.
4. Beecher HK, Todd DP. A study of the deaths associated with anesthesia and surgery: based on a study of 599,548 anesthesia in ten institutions 1948–1952, inclusive. Ann Surg 1954;140(1):2–34.
5. Cooper JB, Newbower RS, Kitz RJ. An analysis of major errors and equipment failures in anesthesia management: considerations for prevention and detection. Anesthesiology 1984;60:34–42.
6. Lowe A, Jones RW, Harrison MJ. The graphical presentation of decision support information in an intelligent anesthesia monitor. Artif Intell Med 2001;22:173–91.
7. Bovill JG. Alarm systems. Baillidre's clinical. Anesthesiology 1990;4(1):193–200.
8. Meredith C, Edworthy J. Are there too many alarms in the intensive are unit? An overview of the problems. J Adv Nurs 1995;21:15–20.
9. Imhoff M, Kuhls S, Gather U, et al. Smart alarms from medical devices in the OR and ICU. Best Pract Res Clin Anaesthesiol 2009;23:39–50.
10. McIntyre J. Ergonomics: anesthetics' use of auditory alarms in the operating room. Int J Clin Monit Comput 1985;2:47–55.
11. Blum JM, Tremper KK. Alarms in the intensive care unit: too much of a good thing is dangerous: is it time to add some intelligence to alarms? Crit Care Med 2010; 38(2):702–3.

12. Chambrin MC, Ravaux P, Calvelo-Aros D. Multicentric study of monitoring alarms in the adult intensive care unit (ICU): a descriptive analysis. Intensive Care Med 1999;25(12):1360–6.
13. Momtahan K, Tansley B. An ergonomic analysis of the auditory alarm signals in the operating room and recovery room. Canadian Acoustics 1989;17(3):93.
14. Meijler A. Automation in anesthesia–a relief? Berlin: Springer-Verlag; 1987. p. 23–4.
15. Kestin I, Miller B, Lockhart C. Auditory alarms during anesthesia monitoring. Anesthesiology 1988;69:106–9.
16. O'Carroll T. Survey of alarms in an intensive therapy unit. Anaesthesia 1986;41:742–4.
17. Lawless ST. Crying wolf: false alarms in a pediatric intensive care unit. Crit Care Med 1994;22(6):981–5.
18. Chambrin M. Alarms in the intensive care unit: how can the number of false alarms be reduced? Crit Care 2001;5(4):184–8.
19. Imhoff M, Kuhls S, Gather U. Clinical relevance of alarms from patient monitors. Crit Care Med 2007;34:A62.
20. Dear G, Panten R, Lubarsky D. Operating room information systems. Semin Anesth Perioperat Med Pain 1999;18(4):322–33.
21. Berner ES, Detmer DE, Simborg D. Will the wave finally break? A brief view of the adoption of electronic medical records in the United States. J Am Med Inform Assoc 2005;12(1):3–7.
22. Osborn JJ. Computers in critical care medicine: promises and pitfalls. Crit Care Med 1982;10:807–10.
23. Gunasekaran S. EMR design: when it comes to healthcare granularity, conceiving and deciding upon design is serious business. Healthc Inform 2007;24(12):44.
24. Patel VL, Shortliffe EH, Stefanelli M, et al. The coming age of artificial intelligence in medicine. Artif Intell Med 2009;46:5–17.
25. Stevenson KB, Barbera J, Moore JW. Understanding keys to successful implementation of electronic decision support in rural hospitals: analysis of a pilot study for antimicrobial prescribing. Am J Med Qual 2005;20(6):313–8.
26. Wadhwa R, Fridsma DB, Saul MI, et al. Analysis of a failed clinical decision support system for management of congestive heart failure. In: Proceedings of the Symposium of the American Medical Informatics Association. Phoenix; 2008. p. 773–7.
27. Toth-Pal E. Implementing a clinical decision-support system in practice: a qualitative analysis of influencing attitudes and characteristics among general practitioners. Inform Health Soc Care 2008;33(1):39–54.
28. van Melle W. MYCIN: a knowledge-based consultation program for infection disease diagnosis. Int J Man Mach Stud 1978;10:313–22.
29. Wolfram DA. An appraisal of INTERNIST-1. Artif Intell Med 1995;7:93–116.
30. Weiss SM, Kulikowski CA, Amarel S. A model-based method for computer-aided medical decision making. Artif Intel 1978;11:145–72.
31. Phillips J. Clinical alarms: complexity and common sense. Surg Clin North Am 2006;18(2):145.
32. Tsien CL, Fackler JC. Poor prognosis for existing monitors in the intensive care unit. Crit Care Med 1997;25(4):614.
33. Peek N, Goud R, Abu-Hanna A. Application of statistical process control methods to monitor guideline adherence: a case study. In: Proceedings of the Symposium of the American Medical Informatics Association. Phoenix; 2008. p. 581–5.
34. Yourman L, Concato J, Agostini JV. Use of computer decision support interventions to improve medication prescribing in older adults: a systematic review. Am J Geriatr Pharmacother 2008;6(2):119–29.

35. Wolfstadt JI. The effect of computerized physician order entry with clinical decision support on the rates of adverse drug events: a systematic review. J Gen Intern Med 2008;23(4):451–8.

36. Isern D, Sanchez D, Moreno A. Agents applied in health care: a review. Int J Med Inform 2010;79:145–66.

37. Gennari JH, Musen MA, Fergerson RW, et al. The evolution of protege: an environment for knowledge-based systems development. Int J Hum Comput Stud 2003;58:89–123.

38. Singh S, Ismail B, Haron F, et al. Architecture of agent-based healthcare intelligent assistant on grid environment. In: Liew K, Shen H, See S, et al, editors. Lecture Notes in Computer Science: Parallel and Distributed Computing: Applications and Technologies, vol. 3320. Berlin (Heidelberg): Springer; 2005. p. 58–61.

39. González-Vélez H, Mier M, Julià-Sapé M, et al. Health Agents: distributed multi-agent brain tumor diagnosis and prognosis. Appl Intell 2009;30(3):191–202.

40. Koutkias V, Chouvarda I, Maglaveras N. A multi-agent system enhancing home-care health services for chronic disease management. IEEE Trans Inf Technol Biomed 2005;9(4):528–37.

41. Cervantes L, Lee Y, Yang H, et al. Agent-based intelligent decision support for the home healthcare environment. In: Szczuka M, Howard D, Slezak D, et al, editors. Lecture Notes in Computer Science: Advances in Hybrid Information Technology, vol. 4413. Berlin (Heidelberg): Springer; 2007. p. 414–24.

42. Chen C, Kruger GH, Blum JM, et al. Reactive agent and visualization system for anesthesia support in the operating room. In: Callaos N, Chu H, Tremante A, editors. Proceedings of the International Conference on Engineering and Meta-Engineering. International Institute of Informatics and Systemics. Florida, 2010.

43. Dahaba AA. Procalcitonin for early prediction of survival outcome in postoperative critically ill patients with severe sepsis. Br J Anaesth 2006;97(4):503–8.

Enhancing Point of Care Vigilance Using Computers

Paul St. Jacques, MD*, Brian Rothman, MD

KEYWORDS

• Informatics • Vigilance • Safety • Perioperative • Surgery

For years medicine has lagged behind other disciplines in the adoption of information technology. Instead, the community had relied on manual and paper processes for documentation, using computers only for systems such as laboratory and billing. Recent events identifying wide-ranging problems in safety and efficiency in medical practice are changing that status. The community now looks to apply lessons related to automation and computerization that were learned in other industries to facilitate change and improvement in medicine.

Computer technology is now being incorporated into medical practice at record pace. However, this technology is frequently implemented as a solution rather than as a tool to achieve a certain goal. In this article, the authors review how the implementation of informatics tools in the perioperative arena can provide information to practitioners to potentially enhance their ability to conduct safe and vigilant care to patients both in their immediate vicinity and across the operating suite. The authors also examine how advanced decision support algorithms may be used with message delivery systems to synthesize and deliver just-in-time information to the perioperative clinician.

SAFETY AND VIGILANCE

For decades, the practice of anesthesiology has defined itself as a leader and advocate for patient safety. An analysis done in 1978 of 359 preventable anesthesia-related accidents revealed that 82% involved human error.[1] Most frequently, these errors were associated with inadequate communication, lack of precaution, or distraction.[1] Almost 3 decades later, communication failures continue to be a source of significant error in the operating room (OR)[2] despite numerous developments in

Paul St. Jacques, MD, is an inventor of the Vanderbilt Perioperative Information Management system and is a minority equity holder and consultant to Acuitec, LLC, Birmingham, AL, USA. Brian Rothman, MD, has no relevant financial disclosures.
Department of Anesthesiology, Vanderbilt University School of Medicine, 1301 Medical Center Drive, 4648 The Vanderbilt Clinic, Nashville, TN 37237, USA
* Corresponding author.
E-mail address: Paul.stjacques@vanderbilt.edu

Anesthesiology Clin 29 (2011) 505–519
doi:10.1016/j.anclin.2011.05.008
1932-2275/11/$ – see front matter © 2011 Elsevier Inc. All rights reserved.

monitoring technology, pharmacology, and clinical practice, which have produced significant declines in surgical patient morbidity and mortality over the same period.

The study and advancement of patient safety has not been confined to anesthesiology. Although anesthesiology has always had an internal focus on safety, the external community has also produced an increased level of scrutiny for medical errors and adverse events caused by medical care.[3] As seen in the previously mentioned studies, the same theme holds true in the landmark report "To Err is Human." The report describes how many of these events may be preventable through the design of systems that focus on communication, training, and better situational awareness.[3]

Information technology is a frequently used asset when looking at methodology for improving safety and reducing costs of health care[4] and can improve safety in several ways. For example, computer systems may prevent errors by providing information, which averts an error or leads to the correction of an error-prone state before a morbidity or mortality event.[5] The same systems can also provide retrospective information related to adverse events and guide future improvement efforts.[5] Error prevention can come in many forms. One such form, simply providing access to retrieve stored computerized information that is otherwise not readily available on paper records, produces significant benefits in reducing repeat testing and increases time efficiencies. Beyond this type of basic information retrieval, information systems can provide additional information to practitioners such as laboratory value ranges, drug adjustment calculations in computerized order entry systems, or potential adverse drug interactions.[4] Beyond such descriptive information, clinical course adjustments can be made. For example, general medical practice uses information systems to ensure that best practice clinical pathways are followed. Modeling ideal pathways for clinicians to follow to manage chronic diseases such as diabetes is an example.[4]

Vigilance is the careful attention to a particular task. It is of paramount importance for ensuring safety in anesthesiology. Vigilance for anesthesiologists in the OR is close attentiveness to the status of the patient. This vigilance is achieved through close physical observation of the patient, monitoring technology, and the OR environment, in general, including the activities of the surgical and nursing teams. The importance of vigilance for the safety of patients undergoing surgery has been heavily reported. Studies have found that adverse outcomes and events are not usually related to the mechanical failure of equipment used in the OR. A study by Cooper and colleagues[6] showed that in 1089 critical incidents, only 4% were attributable to equipment failure. The same study cited human error as the dominant factor and identified key areas of training, supervision, and improved monitoring as the components necessary for improving safety.[6] A landmark report by Weinger and Englund[7] went further to define human factors and ergonomics as significant contributors to OR safety and the propensity for human error. The investigators examined several components, including work environment, human components, and systems/equipment. The findings of this study were that despite good rationale for automating complex systems such as the OR suite, the automation would not in and of itself lead to improved performance and that such developments would need to be studied to examine their effect on outcome.[7]

The OR presents many challenges to maintaining vigilance toward the primary task of monitoring response to changes in patient condition and surgical progress. The OR is a noisy environment, and tasks are subject to interruption. Task interruption has been identified as a potential cause of lapses of safety in the OR.[8] In the complex OR environment, interference of vigilance can come from multiple sources, such as equipment, surgical and nursing staff related to the procedure in progress, and external to the OR in the form of pagers, phone calls, and discussions with other staff. This finding is similar to studies of the aviation model that show interruptions and distractions can lead to errors in the performance of safety checks.[9] Additional human factors such as fatigue have also been studied and found to contribute to a decreased level of detection of changes in monitored variables in an experimental setting.[10] Summarizing these studies reveals, not surprisingly, that the OR is a complex environment with large number of distracting events, with potentially poor ergonomics, and operated by practitioners who are subject to limitations in their ability to maintain vigilance. From this vantage point, the authors examine how information technology is currently being used, how future developments may be used to improve patient safety through the synthesis of needed information, and the delivery of that information in a streamlined manner that minimizes noise and maximizes benefit to the patient and practitioner.

INFORMATION TECHNOLOGY

There are many examples of the use of information technology in the OR suite. Clinical documentation systems record events, procedures, medications, and other items in a patient's care. Charge capture systems ensure that patients are not charged for items that are not needed while ensuring that facilities have proper accounting of items that are used during a procedure. Electronic digital radiology systems have replaced traditional radiographs and have brought new dimensions to capture, storage, retrieval, and display of medical images. Even more complex systems such as integrated endoscopy and stereotactic guidance systems are widely used.

To better understand the background of documentation systems, a graphical representation of a complete perioperative medical record system may incorporate many interfaced subsystems and applications as shown in **Fig. 1**. Institutions have adopted clinical information systems for the perioperative area very slowly, particularly for anesthesiology.[11] Many have implemented systems that do not contain all the components needed and are designed to only handle very basic documentation tasks of current care. Some of the more advanced systems may offer access to stored electronic medical records or incorporate the function of tracking patients' progress through the surgical suite. Patient tracking may be accomplished through manual or electronic means such as radio frequency identification (RFID) or location systems.[12] At an even higher level, other systems provide more value-added functions, such as integration of the bedside patient monitor data, other medical device data, and even video to provide a more complete analysis of patient care.[13] Systems with a broader suite-wide scope provide information about multiple patients. These systems incorporate electronic scheduling boards or Web sites that provide the distributed knowledge of the constantly changing OR schedule. This information is used by the various care teams in the surgical suite. An example of an electronic schedule board is shown in **Fig. 2**. Other indicators of patient status may accompany basic patient information, which includes current patient location, the state of documentation completeness, and any missing surgical consents or postoperative orders. From any location, staff can easily see what information is available and take the appropriate action based on what they learn from the display.

The future holds promise for even broader applications. Expanding the limits beyond the walls of a single hospital, information technology is now being used to provide remote telepresence and clinical expertise in remote locations. For example, a 2004 report showed how technology could be used to remotely monitor vital signs

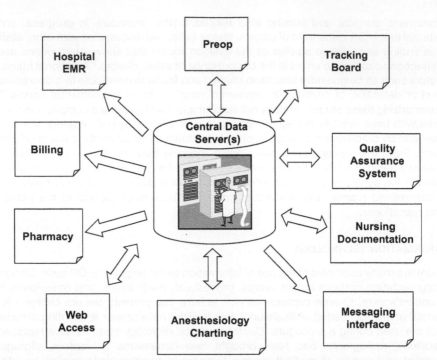

Fig. 1. A perioperative information management system (PIMS) may consist of several inter-faced related systems tracking documentation of care; physiologic parameters, such as vital signs from bedside monitors; data from laboratory systems; and patient tracking systems. PIMS may then produce additional data for other hospital systems such as billing, pharmacy, and quality assurance. A PIMS database is typically centered on a computer server or series of servers held in a centralized data center. EMR, Electronic Medical Record.

data transmitted from a surgery in Ecuador to a collaborative site in the United States.[14] Even more extreme examples using telepresence robots have been described that enable remote practitioners to virtually visit patients and carry on 2-way audio-visual conversations.[15] Through such a system, a consultant is able to communicate with remote OR staff from a control station. Full-duplex audio and video facilitate communication via a remotely controlled mobile robotic device.[16]

SITUATIONAL AWARENESS

Situational awareness is the perception of environmental elements, the comprehension of their meaning, and the prediction of a future state based on those elements and their meaning. In other words, situational awareness is the understanding and awareness of what is happening around you.[17] It requires 2 components: information and practitioner vigilance to that information. In the context of anesthesiology, this awareness may consist of what is happening in the OR and the entire surgical care.

In addition to the OR, elements of patient care in the preoperative holding room and postanesthesia care unit (PACU) are also within the domain of the anesthesiologist. **Fig. 3** shows that when the preoperative holding area and PACU census is considered, a single anesthesiologist may have some level of responsibility to several patients at any given time in addition to the needs and status of any patient in the OR (see

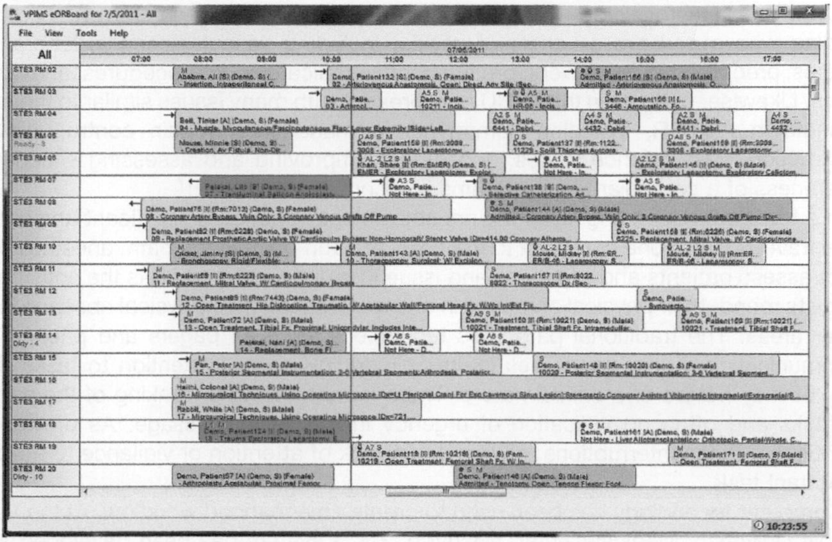

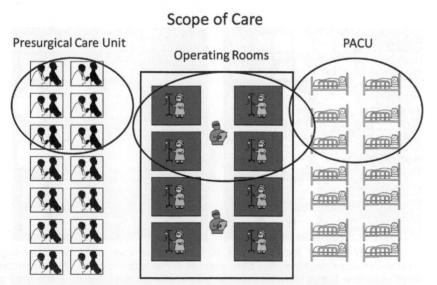

Fig. 2. An electronic schedule board provides access to current scheduling information to perioperative staff. Data presented may include patient- and procedure-specific information, information about patient readiness for surgery, information about room set up status, and case start or completion delays. Using this information, managers can project room occupancy and arrange the schedule to maximize efficiency while clinicians can use the same information to obtain critical patient information. (*Courtesy of* Acuitec, LLC, Birmingham, AL, USA; with permission.)

Scope of Care

Presurgical Care Unit

Operating Rooms

PACU

Fig. 3. The situational awareness of anesthesiologists must consider not only the patient currently in any OR for which they have responsibility but also those patients who are preparing to have surgery and those who are recovering in the PACU.

Fig. 3). The anesthesiologist may be responsible for patients in the preoperative holding who may have a variety of needs, including vascular access, laboratory studies, preoperative paperwork, preanesthetic medications or procedures, and other items. Likewise, patients in the PACU may present with many issues similar to those in patients in the OR, including hemodynamic management, pain control, airway obstruction, fluid balance issues, and others. Improving and assessing situational awareness of a particular team or teams is a complex analysis.[17]

In a traditional operating suite, the anesthesiologist spends a significant amount of time traveling from one care area to the next. At each point in the path, anesthesiologists assess patients and situations and issue instructions for care. As the anesthesiologists round, their physical presence in one area means their physical absence in all other areas. The traditional path uses technology such as pagers and phones for communication. These modalities interrupt workflow to call attention to tasks that may or may not be of a critical nature. There is no queuing or ranking of the pages or tasks and often no indication of urgency in the initial message. As previously mentioned, these interruptions may lead to a lack of attention or vigilance to a more important task.

Computer technology has been used to create an enhanced workflow. At the Vanderbilt University Medical Center, Nashville, TN, a system has been developed and implemented that integrates information from multiple sources and delivers that information to the clinician via handheld computers and communication devices, including cellular devices and pagers (Fig. 4).

This system integrates data from the perioperative information management systems. The primary information management systems are used to schedule surgical cases, track patient flow, and document nursing and anesthesiology care in all stages of surgery from preoperative evaluation to the PACU. Laboratory data and live video from cameras located in each OR and in the PACU are additional data sources integrated into the stream. Physiologic data, such as vital signs, are interfaced from bedside monitors and other sources and presented as waveforms and trends. Data

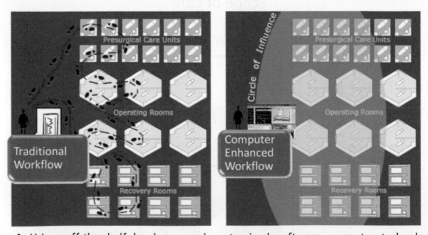

Fig. 4. Using off-the-shelf hardware and customized software computer technology, a computer-enhanced workflow has been created for anesthesiologists. This computer-enhanced workflow brings important clinical information to the clinician in the form of integrated displays on handheld computers and communication devices. Thus, the clinicians are able to expand their situational awareness to an entire OR suite and may be better able to more efficiently serve the needs of the patients under their care.

are fed via Ethernet to a series of servers, which analyze and format the data for presentation. Reformatted data are then returned to the clinicians via a wired or wireless network to either desktop or handheld computers (**Fig. 5**).

In addition to reformatted data, the system can provide text messages via pagers or cell phones. The messages include physiologic notices, such as blood pressures or heart rates, out of a set range and status messages, such as patients arriving to the holding room or cases closing. Clinicians are required to initially access the application to subscribe to the data feeds and messages for specific ORs and patients. In the subscription process, the clinician can subscribe to a set template of values and customize the messages for any particular patient. The template initially includes values that are global for the department, but each clinician may customize the template to match his or her clinical practice. Clinicians can further individualize the messages to match the unique needs of an individual patient.

The user interface of this system is designed to present a graphic OR suite schedule, similar to what is displayed on a larger electronic OR board. The graphic schedule representation allows for a better understanding of the overall status of the operating suite than does a list of cases. The touch screen interface allows the user to select any particular case for further examination. Selecting a case shows a full-screen integrated display of patient monitor waveform data, vital signs trends, live video and case, and demographic information on the full-scale workstation (**Fig. 6**). A multiple-view mode allows the user to view simultaneous video from up to 4 operating areas, with the most recent set of vital signs displayed below each video

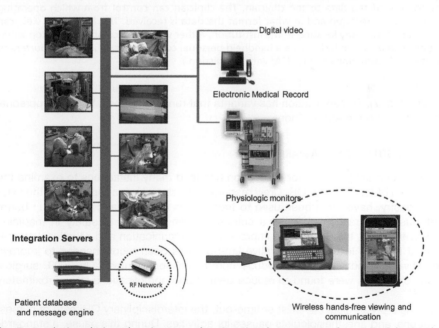

Fig. 5. A solution designed to improve the situational awareness of anesthesiologists by aggregating information from a plurality of monitors and data sources and video cameras. The system integrates the information via data processing servers, delivering that information via a wireless computer device. In using this system, the anesthesiologist can selectively receive information from one or several operating and PACU locations. A messaging system accompanies the data integration system so that notifications from physiologic or process changes can be delivered to the user in an automated fashion. RF, radio frequency.

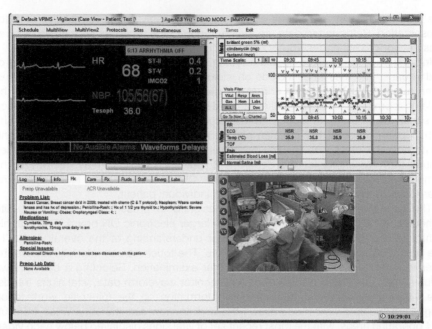

Fig. 6. The informatics system gathers data from multiple sources and presents an integrated view of the data to the clinician. The clinician can control from which operating site the data is received and in what format the data is received. This integrated view can be obtained from any location in the institution, either via a fixed computer desktop workstation or in a mobile fashion via a handheld personal computer or an iPhone. (*Courtesy of* Acuitec, LLC, Birmingham, AL, USA; with permission.)

stream (**Fig. 7**). The application has variants that run on handheld Windows personal computers and the Apple iPhone.

OR LEVEL SITUATIONAL AWARENESS

The focus on safety and error prevention has lead many institutions to examine the interaction of teams in the OR. Crew management strategies, adopted from the aviation industry, have often been used to train teams of physicians and staff in better methods of interaction to foster a culture and environment of safety in medicine and, specifically, the OR.[18,19] To improve the communication and situational awareness at the staff level, a preoperative time-out has been recommended to improve proactive communication and reduce communication failures.[20] In 2009, surgical safety checklists were found to reduce deaths and complications by approximately 50%.[21]

During a presurgical checklist or time-out, the interdisciplinary OR team of nurses, surgeons, and anesthesiologists pauses its activities. During this pause, a standardized checklist is read and often compared with written information on a whiteboard in the OR. Checklist items include patient identification, surgical procedure and laterality, patient allergies, and so forth. However, the information is only as good as what it is being compared with. Manual whiteboards may be prone to error, such as information that is copied incorrectly, information leftover from a previous case, or information that is absent entirely.

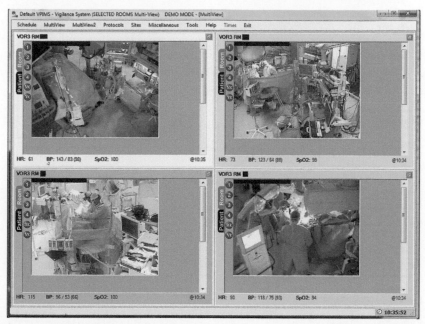

Fig. 7. The same integration software provides a view to as many as 4 simultaneous video feeds on the fixed or mobile handheld device. Video feeds are selectable by the user and include a presentation of the most recent set of vital signs received from the bedside monitor. (*Courtesy of* Acuitec, LLC, Birmingham, AL, USA; with permission.)

Electronic resources can assist in accurately providing the key patient's data elements for use during the presurgical checklist. By replacing the manual whiteboard with an electronic whiteboard coupled to an electronic documentation system, it becomes possible for the comparator information used during the checklist to accurately reflect the patient's medical record and surgical schedule. A large liquid crystal display (LCD) placed on the OR wall where it is in full view of the OR staff has been used for this function. The LCD board is formatted to display the key information needed, and it updates itself on the patient's exit from the OR. During the time-out checklist, each element of the checklist is highlighted so that all in the OR are attentive and are enabled to agree or disagree before the next element being verified (**Fig. 8**). At the completion of the time-out, notification is displayed and the board reverts to a mode that displays case information and pertinent staff and scheduling information to better assist team communication and efficiency.

OPERATING SUITE SITUATIONAL AWARENESS

Situational awareness must extend beyond the OR. Technology can enable OR managers and avoid problems such as tracking patients through the process of surgery. In a traditional system, patient tracking requires the use of manual updates to pen or grease board-based whiteboards. Generally, these boards are located in key management areas such as the OR board and holding room or PACU desks. The only way to determine a patient's location using this method is to physically visit each location and review the whiteboard in that area, assuming that the whiteboard is up-to-date and accurate. This type of system does not notify staff of changes in status or schedules. It may lead to inefficiencies with resources being misdirected toward

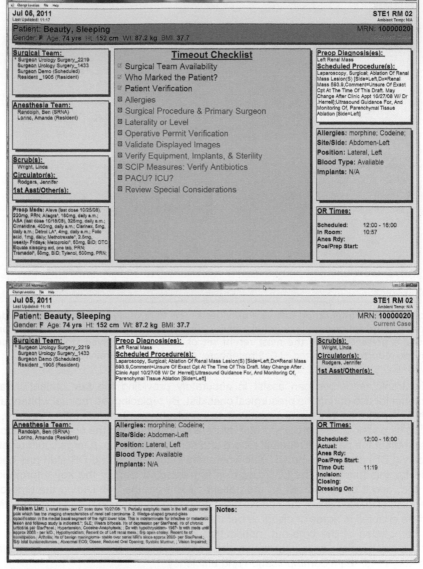

Fig. 8. An electronic checklist whiteboard is displayed on a large LCD panel in the OR to assist in team situational awareness and safety. The top panel shows the configuration of the board during the surgical safety checklist. After checklist completion, the board displays key patient, case, and staff information as shown in the lower panel. (*Courtesy of* Acuitec, LLC, Birmingham, AL, USA; with permission.)

surgeries that have changed time or location or toward patients who are no longer in the documented area.

An electronic scheduling and tracking system can alleviate many of those issues. Electronic schedule boards are designed in such a way that information is available from any location in which the schedule board software runs. Staffs no longer need to travel to different sites to keep up-to-date on the current state of the schedule and each patient on the schedule. It is also possible to automate changes in patient status by linking the scheduling board to the documentation system such that users enter changes to patient status as a part of the normal documentation of clinical care. Taking this one step further, it is even possible to couple the electronic information system to indoor locations systems using modalities such as RFID, infrared, and ultrasound to automatically update patient location. One design provides information to the clinicians about patients being brought to the wrong location by coupling room-level electronic patient location to a schedule/location database and notifying clinicians of any mismatches.[12] Even without any additional technology, it has been shown that an event such as the initiation of patient monitoring can be detected electronically through a software interface and used as an indicator of a patient entering an OR.[22] These solutions represent an improvement in situational awareness at a macrolevel. The anesthesiologist can have a better understanding of the status of each patient in the OR suite without relying on a manual process in a distant location.

COMMUNICATION

As previously mentioned, issues related to communication are associated with many adverse events.[3] Improving communication in a way that enhances the practitioner's ability to maintain vigilance to important detail is a critical factor in systems design. Traditional communication methodologies require a clinician in one area, for example, a nurse anesthetist in an OR, to identify a pattern or suspected problem before triggering a communication event. That person then typically retrieves a pager number, dials the number, enters a return number, and waits for a return call to transfer the information. Under ideal circumstances, this communication is slow. A typical pager-initiated communication event takes an average of 118 seconds.[23] Other modalities of communication such as voice over Internet protocol or instant on cellular may reduce the communication latency and failure rate.[23] However, these technologies are not yet widely deployed in the OR. Future development not only will computerize the content of the communications made in the OR but also may direct that information to the appropriate personnel. Situations may call for immediate action from the closest provider or may allow for a longer response time from a more distant provider with more knowledge of or responsibility for a certain patient. For example, Botsis and colleagues[24] describe a context-aware communication system that automatically routes calls and pages to particular devices depending on device status and proximity to the needed response. It is possible that in the future when someone calls for help, the call will automatically be routed not only to the physician who is requested but also to the person who can best respond. This ideal responder could be determined through a computerized analysis of provider skill sets coupled with specific information of a highly emergent situation.

SMART SYSTEMS AND DECISION SUPPORT

Automated messages are pieces of information that are sent to a clinician without any user triggering or additional input. An example would be a notification that a patient has entered a room being delivered to a wireless pager. Clinicians can receive this message and judge the timing of their entry to the OR to minimize interruptions and waiting times for a patient who is not yet ready for induction. These messages can be delivered via software to a handheld computer device such as an Apple iPhone or iPod Touch device via cellular network or Wi-Fi. Using one of these handheld devices and software, a clinician can receive a variety of messages. When needed, they respond to those messages using either a preconfigured response or a specific response created at that time (**Fig. 9**). The clinician can also choose to obtain additional information regarding the message by viewing specific patient data such as vital signs trends or live video streams from the location where the page originated.

Information technology can be used to bring existing data to clinicians. This technology potentially improves clinicians' ability to proactively respond to a situation more effectively compared with not receiving the information or receiving the information in a manner that does not enhance their ability to prioritize tasks and maintain vigilance to a primary task or set of tasks. However, computerized analysis of data can provide more than information relay. Systems can be designed that analyze and synthesize new information. This newly synthesized information can then be delivered to and used by the clinician to enhance care. Numerous examples of this have been demonstrated in the literature.

Prophylactic presurgical antibiotic administration is a commonly omitted yet routine task. It serves as a prime example of how the application of decision support systems benefits patient outcomes. Administration of antibiotics before surgical incision for the prevention of surgical site infection is a task that has achieved national significance. It is well known that failure to administer antibiotics before skin incision leads to increased infection risks.[25] However, what is less well known is that because of clinician distraction, interruptions, and other factors, this task was previously frequently forgotten in the course of surgical care. Computerized systems have been developed that act as watchdogs, providing reminders to monitor the course of the anesthetic care and provide a message to the provider that the antibiotics are due. This system has been developed in different information systems as a pop-up reminder, a step on an annotated care path, or a separate visual indicator on the documentation computer screen.[26,27] Using these systems, compliance with the standard protocol was found to increase to greater than 90%.

More sophisticated analyses can also be conducted in which databases of past anesthetic care records are electronically reviewed to generate predictions of negative outcomes. Development of expert systems and rule-based systems is not a new concept. In 2007, Meyer and colleagues[13] described the use of artificial neural

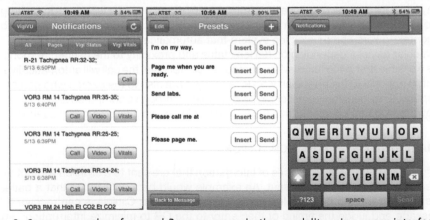

Fig. 9. Screen examples of a novel 2-way communication modality using pager interfaces recreated on a handheld computer device. The pages are delivered by the standard pager messaging system, with a redirection at the server level to the handheld computer (*left panel*). The user has the option of responding to the page with a preset (*center panel*) or custom message (*right panel*) and can also choose to obtain more information such as a review of vital signs trends or live video from the location from which the page was sent.

networks to approach multivariate monitoring and pattern recognition. The investigators conclude that greater utility can be achieved when data from multiple systems was integrated and analyzed together compared with what could be achieved from the analysis of one output, even a trended output from a single monitor. In later work, this concept was used to create a system that predicted light anesthesia through detecting changes in computer-filtered data from heart rate and blood pressure monitors.[28]

Not all decision support and expert systems involve monitoring technologies. Vast databases of information are created during the surgical care process. These databases can be analyzed for outcomes data based on individual patient characteristics. One such study has shown that a computerized database scan of 50,000 anesthetics for indicators of impossible mask ventilation revealed key factors in this rare event.[29] In another study, a computerized database scan was undertaken in a review of 65,000 anesthetics to examine for risk factors for postoperative renal failure.[30] It is a straightforward process to translate this type of research to a system that actively scans each patient's data record before or during surgery and predicts what negative outcomes are likely to occur. It could then forewarn the clinical staff of those potential outcomes so that preventative steps can be taken. The communication systems the authors have described can then relay this information to the clinician based on a combination of clinical and surgical contexts.

It is easy to predict that in the future, an expert computerized system will examine the current state of a patient undergoing surgery for any deviation from the normal care process. The computer would then compare that deviation to other patients who have had similar characteristics and similar deviations. It would analyze and weigh the deviation based on the type of surgery, the stage of surgery, and the duration of the deviation. The system then warns the clinician of a potential adverse outcome and possibly even suggests steps to avoid the adverse outcome. Similar systems have been in place in other industries such as aviation with great success.[31]

IMPACT ON OUTCOMES

Despite significant work on the development of information technology–related systems to support the safety of patients in the OR, little advanced work has been undertaken to prove that these systems have the ability to improve the vigilance or situational awareness of the practitioner or improve the outcome of the patient through a reduction in short- or long-term morbidity and mortality. However, financial studies have supported the use of decision support in terms of providing documentation reminders to clinicians to enable improvements in billing accuracy and charge capture. Spring and colleagues[32] has shown a marked reduction in nonbillable charts as a result of an intervention that automatically scanned computerized records and notified physicians of incomplete or missing data. On a smaller scale, attention to billing individual procedures has benefited from an electronic reminder system in which supervising clinician documentation of arterial line procedures is prompted. It resulted in improved billing and collections for those procedures.[33] The lack of outcomes studies showing patient benefit in terms of morbidity and mortality should not detract from the development of systems that benefit vigilance and safety. A striking example of this concept can be seen in an article that examines the benefits of parachutes in preventing death and major trauma.[34]

SUMMARY

Vigilance and situational awareness remain paramount to patient safety. Coupled with advances in communications, new generations of informatics systems will enhance patient safety and efficiency at the levels of the patient, the OR, and the OR suite. Information provided by these systems will not be in the traditional alarm- or alert-type format. New information will be synthesized from existing raw data and historical databases and will be context specific and rich in value. The demands of an ever-enlarging need for medical services in an environment that is driving toward cost-efficiency and improvements in outcomes will drive the need for further development and implementation.

REFERENCES

1. Cooper JB, Newbower RS, Long CD, et al. Preventable anesthesia mishaps: a study of human factors. Qual Saf Health Care 2002;11(3):277.
2. Lingard L, Espin S, Whyte S, et al. Communication failures in the operating room: an observational classification of recurrent types and effects. BMJ 2004;13(5):330.
3. Kohn LT, Corrigan J, Donaldson MS. To err is human: building a safer health system. Washington, DC: Natl Academy Pr; 2000.
4. Hillestad R, Bigelow J, Bower A, et al. Can electronic medical record systems transform health care? Potential health benefits, savings, and costs. Health Aff 2005;24(5):1103.
5. Bates DW, Gawande AA. Improving safety with information technology. N Engl J Med 2003;348(25):2526–34.
6. Cooper JB, Newbower RS, Kitz RJ. An analysis of major errors and equipment failures in anesthesia management: considerations for prevention and detection. Anesthesiology 1984;60(1):34.
7. Weinger MB, Englund CE. Ergonomic and human factors affecting anesthetic vigilance and monitoring performance in the operating room environment. Anesthesiology 1990;73(5):995–1021.
8. Healey AN, Sevdalis N, Vincent CA. Measuring intra-operative interference from distraction and interruption observed in the operating theatre. Ergonomics 2006; 49(5):589–604.
9. Latorella KA. Investigating interruptions: implications for flightdeck performance. Hanover (MD): NASA Center for AeroSpace Information; 1999.
10. Denisco RA, Drummond JN, Gravenstein JS. The effect of fatigue on the performance of a simulated anesthetic monitoring task. J Clin Monit 1987;3(1):22–4.
11. Halbeis E, Christoph B, Epstein RH, et al. Adoption of anesthesia information management systems by academic departments in the United States. Anesth Analg 2008;107(4):1323.
12. Sandberg WS, Hakkinen M, Egan M, et al. Automatic detection and notification of "wrong patient–wrong location" errors in the operating room. Surg Innov 2005; 12(3):253.
13. Meyer MA, Levine WC, Egan MT, et al. A computerized perioperative data integration and display system. Int J Comput Assist Radiol Surg 2007;2(3):191–202.
14. Cone SW, Gehr L, Hummel R, et al. Case report of remote anesthetic monitoring using telemedicine. Anesth Analg 2004;98(2):386–8.
15. Smith CD, Skandalakis JE. Remote presence proctoring by using a wireless remote-control videoconferencing system. Surg Innov 2005;12(2):139.
16. Agarwal R, Levinson AW, Allaf M, et al. The RoboConsultant: telementoring and remote presence in the operating room during minimally invasive urologic surgeries using a novel mobile robotic interface. Urology 2007;70(5):970–4.
17. Wright MC. Objective measures of situation awareness in a simulated medical environment. Qual Saf Health Care 2004;13(Suppl 1):i65–71.

18. James M, Otten T, Poggi M, et al. The challenge of changing roles and improving surgical care now: crew resource management approach. Am Surg 2006;72(11): 1082–7.

19. Dunn EJ, Mills PD, Neily J, et al. Medical team training: applying crew resource management in the Veterans Health Administration. Jt Comm J Qual Patient Saf 2007;33(6):317–25.

20. Lingard L, Regehr G, Orser B, et al. Evaluation of a preoperative checklist and team briefing among surgeons, nurses, and anesthesiologists to reduce failures in communication. Arch Surg 2008;143(1):12.

21. Haynes AB, Weiser TG, Berry WR, et al. A surgical safety checklist to reduce morbidity and mortality in a global population. N Engl J Med 2009;360(5):491–9.

22. Xiao Y, Hu P, Hu H, et al. An algorithm for processing vital sign monitoring data to remotely identify operating room occupancy in real-time. Anesth Analg 2005; 101(3):823–9.

23. Jacques PS, France DJ, Pilla M, et al. Evaluation of a hands-free wireless communication device in the perioperative environment. Telemed J E Health 2006;12(1): 42–9.

24. Botsis T, Solvoll T, Scholl J, et al. Context-aware systems for mobile communication in healthcare: a user oriented approach. In: Proceedings of the 7th Conference on 7th WSEAS International Conference on Applied Informatics and Communications-Volume 7. Los Alamos (CA): IEEE Computer Society Press; 2007. p. 69–74.

25. Bratzler DW, Houck PM. Antimicrobial prophylaxis for surgery: an advisory statement from the National Surgical Infection Prevention Project. Clin Infect Dis 2004; 38:1706–15.

26. Jacques PS, Sanders N, Patel N, et al. Improving timely surgical antibiotic prophylaxis redosing administration using computerized record prompts. Surg Infect 2005;6(2):215–21.

27. O'Reilly M, Talsma AN, VanRiper S, et al. An anesthesia information system designed to provide physician-specific feedback improves timely administration of prophylactic antibiotics. Anesth Analg 2006;103(4):908.

28. Krol M, Reich DL. Development of a decision support system to assist anesthesiologists in operating room. J Med Syst 2000;24(3):141–6.

29. Kheterpal S, Han R, Tremper KK, et al. Incidence and predictors of difficult and impossible mask ventilation. Anesthesiology 2006;105(5):885.

30. Kheterpal S, Tremper KK, Englesbe MJ, et al. Predictors of postoperative acute renal failure after noncardiac surgery in patients with previously normal renal function. Anesthesiology 2007;107(6):892.

31. Wilson JR. Faster warnings for safer skies. Aero Am 1990;38(1):30–2 (0740-722 X).

32. Spring SF, Sandberg WS, Anupama S, et al. Automated documentation error detection and notification improves anesthesia billing performance. Anesthesiology 2007;106(1):157.

33. Kheterpal S, Gupta R, Blum JM, et al. Electronic reminders improve procedure documentation compliance and professional fee reimbursement. Anesth Analg 2007;104(3):592.

34. Smith G, Pell JP. Parachute use to prevent death and major trauma related to gravitational challenge: systematic review of randomised controlled trials. BMJ 2003;327(7429):1459.

The Use of Computers for Perioperative Simulation in Anesthesia, Critical Care, and Pain Medicine

Simon Lambden, FRCA[a],*, Bruce Martin, FRCA[b]

KEYWORDS

• Simulation • Computers • Anesthesia

Until recently, medical training has revolved around the apprenticeship model of learning, with junior doctors observing and then performing tasks in real-life situations under decreasing levels of supervision—the so-called see one, do one, teach one method.

Several limitations of the apprenticeship model have always existed, including the ethical challenges of allowing trainees to make mistakes, the balance of optimum patient care and educational requirements, and the interpatient variability that makes no two patient encounters the same.

Recent years have seen several changes in the delivery of health care and training, each making the apprenticeship model a less valid and acceptable tool. These changes include a reduction in junior doctors' hours with a consequent drop in total experience gained over the course of a training program and an increasingly litigious society that requires objective assessment of ability. This shift has coincided with the introduction of competence-based training in some countries, including the United Kingdom, where trainees are expected to show competence in those skills required for their level of training before progressing in their programs.

All of these things have led to an increased interest in the use of simulation as a tool to train and assess both individuals and teams. This article addresses the potential

Dr Martin declares his interest in HeartWorks, IML Ltd as one of the inventors and project directors.

[a] Department of Anaesthesia Critical Care and Pain, University College London Hospitals, 235 Euston Road, London, NW1 2BU, UK

[b] Department of Anaesthesia and Critical Care, The Heart Hospital UCLH NHS Foundation Trust, 16 Westmoreland Street, London, W1G 8PH, UK

* Corresponding author.

E-mail address: simonlambden@doctors.net.uk

benefits of simulation in training, discusses the limitations, and then reviews the different technologies that can be used during training in anesthesia and critical care.

Simulation is the act of mimicking a real object, or process of assuming its appearance or outward qualities.[1] Therefore, the suspension of disbelief is a requirement for simulator use because it is not identical to the actual process being trained or tested.

When effective, the use of simulation confers several benefits. A Best Evidence in Medical Education review in 2005 stated that high-fidelity simulation can facilitate learning through, amongst other things, provision of feedback, repetitive practice, curriculum integration, and the capacity to offer a range of levels of difficulty and clinical conditions in a controlled environment.[2] Simulation training is used at no risk to patients or trainees and mistakes are permitted. Each participant can encounter an identical representation of a particular disease process or problem, which can range from common to rare events based on the requirements of those being trained. Simulation of all kinds may therefore offer a valid additional way to train junior doctors given the increasing pressure on working hours and structured teaching time.

Simulation technologies available to trainers in perioperative care can be broadly divided into three categories: fully immersive simulation, virtual reality (VR), and Web- and computer-based simulation. Each of these will be addressed in turn and their development and potential applications developed.

IMMERSIVE SIMULATION TECHNOLOGY

Fully immersive computer-driven simulation in medicine evolved from simple resuscitation simulators first developed in the early 1960s. Laerdal's Resusci Anne was a simple mechanical model designed for training in the basic skills of resuscitation, the ABC approach, and the simple maneuvers of cardiopulmonary resuscitation.[3] In the mid-1960s, a government-funded project in the United States developed SimOne, a model designed to train anesthesia residents. This was driven by an analog computer and, although advanced for its time, lacked the sophistication and flexibility to possess broad appeal, and therefore only one was ever constructed.[4]

In 1968, a part-task trainer for simulating the examination of the cardiovascular system was demonstrated.[5] "Harvey" and its subsequent evolutions went a long way to show the value of physiologic simulation. This tool was the first for which an evidence base was demonstrated, with medical students showing an improved confidence and ability to detect and interpret clinical findings in actual patients.[6] It has subsequently also been used for continued professional development and assessment in a broad range of both primary and secondary care applications, including the education of nurses, physicians, and family practitioners in examination and identification of cardiovascular pathology.[7-9]

The major changes in the use of immersive simulation came with the advances in the ability of computer programs to model physiologic and pharmacologic systems and rapidly respond to events that occur during the simulation. This advancement led to the near-simultaneous development of several computerized systems, with a much greater degree of realism or fidelity than seen previously. Two of these devices were the Comprehensive Anesthesia Simulation Environment (CASE) series of models developed in Stanford University by Gaba and colleagues.[10] which has subsequently become the MedSim Eagle simulator and the Gainesville Anesthesia Simulator (GAS), which was created in the University of Florida.[11] The CASE series combined operator-driven and physiologic and pharmacologic modeling to drive the responses to participant interventions, with the model displaying a broad range of variable physical findings, from adjustable intubation grade to neuromuscular monitoring with thumb twitch. The MedSim series of simulator products are no longer commercially available, however. Evidence for the efficacy of these systems came from improved trainee confidence and a study stopped early because of participant request. Investigators reported an improved learning curve in clinical assessments in a simulation-trained group compared with a group who underwent conventional training.[12] The authors reported that by the end of the trial period, both groups had reached the same standard.

The GAS system was subsequently licensed and has evolved into one of the most common high-fidelity patient simulators used today in the form of the Human Patient Simulator (Medical Education Technologies Inc, Sarasota, FL, USA). Originally, the GAS system was designed to detect faults in anesthetic machines; however, the addition of a lung model and mannequin made it practical as a training tool particularly for anesthesia because of its ability to model volatile agent uptake and distribution. The subsequent addition of injection recognition software made later versions more autonomous, and following progressive development, the METI system available today offers high fidelity and a relatively hands-off approach, with the simulator able to respond to a broad range of trainee interventions.

Another moderate- to high-fidelity simulator commonly used in immersive training is a direct descendent of the Resuci Anne model of the 1960s. The SimMan and its smaller cousin SimBaby (Laerdal Medical Limited, Orpington, Kent, United Kingdom) are both widely used in simulation training and assessment. These moderate- to high-fidelity simulators combine an air compressor to drive mechanical components following either preprogrammed or real-time entries on a separate controlling computer. A simple interface makes it popular, and subsequent generations have brought an increasing degree of complexity. The most recent SimMan model offers the ability to assess and manage cardiovascular, respiratory, and airway disease with recording of pharmacologic and other interventions through radiofrequency identification, thereby facilitating the feedback process. The SimMan is widely used in the United Kingdom, including in the primary examination of the Fellowship of the Royal College of Anaesthetists during the Objective Structured Clinical Examination component.

The group in Germany developed an alternative approach used to generate intraoperative crisis simulations, the Leiden anesthesia simulator, which combined commercially available airway and vascular access trainers with inexpensive signal generators to produce a simulation environment for use in the operating theater by anesthetic trainees.[13]

This type of simulation training is traditionally delivered in formal simulation centers. These centers are usually built apart from clinical settings and designed to replicate specific environments, such as operating and emergency rooms. Because they are expensive (up to $500,000) and are therefore a relatively scarce resource, many clinicians will have minimal access to these facilities.[14] In addition, most centers train clinicians using single-specialty groups. This loss of the multidisciplinary team and participants acting outside their normal role means that they gain experience that is far removed form clinical reality, and an additional level of buy-in is required by participants during this kind of simulation.

These limitations have seen the rise in recent years of simulation delivered at the point of care. "In situ" simulation has been suggested as a means to deliver training to complete teams with a reduced impact on clinical services. The increasing portability of simulation and audiovisual recording equipment that comes with wireless technology means that training can be undertaken in actual clinical areas, testing systems, and individual and team interactions that are difficult to reproduce in a formal simulation center.[15–17] This kind of training confers the additional advantage that participants need not be removed from clinical duties for days at a time but can undertake training within their working day. Evidence for the benefit of this kind of training comes mainly in the areas of resuscitation, with an American group demonstrating that point-of-care simulation training improved adherence to national guidelines for resuscitation, skill levels, and knowledge retention compared with conventional life support training.[18–20]

In addition to its use to test personnel, point-of-care simulation has also found a role in testing new systems and environments, such as in assessing the safety mechanisms in place in a new location for intraoperative radiotherapy.[21,22]

Limitations of this kind of simulation include a dependence on both the support of management staff and the availability of clinical areas, which may be inconsistent. Also, clinical requirements can disrupt this kind of training in a way that is not encountered in formal training centers.

The integration of immersive simulation training in anesthesia and critical care practice has been patchy, with some investigators suggesting that this is because of a lack of high-quality evidence for the use of these tools.[23] Although immersive simulation training has been widely shown to be popular, be considered realistic, and possess both content and construct validity, evidence is limited as to a direct association between this kind of learning and improved patient outcomes, perhaps partly because of the multifactorial nature of the patient journey and the complexity of the adverse events that they encounter. The possibility exists that a combination of modes of immersive simulation training, each used to exploit their advantages, will lead to greater acceptance and uptake of the tool.

The applications of immersive simulation technology can be broadly divided into two categories, technical and nontechnical skills training. Technical skills are the procedural processes that clinicians undertake each day, ranging from laryngoscopy to central venous catheter insertion. The challenge for simulation is achieving the required level of realism to make technical training a meaningful experience. This function has certainly been achieved in some areas, such as resuscitation, in which the quality of the efforts of participants at chest compression and ventilation can be assessed objectively through the simulator itself.[24] Much of the work in the field of technical skill assessment in simulation has been performed in surgery, but the traditional binary "yes/no" technical assessment tools have been recognized to be an inadequate reflection of an individual's ability in this setting.[25,26]

Nontechnical skills are less tangible but still essential components for anesthesia and critical care practitioners to possess. Responsible for a high proportion of adverse events, these skills include communication with others, decision making, situation awareness, and leadership.[27] In many respects, simulation is extremely well suited to the conduct of this kind of training, a fact recognized by the airline industry and first taken up in medicine by anesthesiologists.[28–30] Both of these groups used it in teaching individuals and teams and in assessing their ability to perform well in crisis situations. In fact, the development of early immersive simulators in anesthesia was with particular reference to their potential use to improve nontechnical skills. Extensive work has been undertaken to develop tools to facilitate assessment of nontechnical performance in the operating room, building on scoring systems originally used in the airline industry to assess performance of air crews in simulated airline emergencies.[31] As a result, Anesthesia Crisis Resource Management has become a widely accepted component of anesthesia training, with many trainees expected to gain experience during crisis situations in the simulator as part of their curriculum.[32] The scoring tools that have been developed for this purpose not only serve as a useful assessment tool but also, perhaps more importantly, facilitate the process of structured feedback, giving trainers a platform to highlight specific areas, such as leadership, decision making, time management, or communication, therefore improving the quality and value of the simulation training experience.

VIRTUAL REALITY

VR offered a novel way for humans and computers to interact. It was first developed in the mid-1960s, but was not named virtual reality until approximately 20 years later. Several classifications have been suggested, although the most widely used is that of immersive and nonimmersive VR. In immersive VR systems, the user is completely integrated into an environment created by a computer. This model may include visual, auditory, olfactory, touch, and force feedback (haptic) sensations. This technology is extremely complex and costly, and therefore the most commonly used form of VR is nonimmersive technology. In these systems, a variable but incomplete interaction occurs between the user and the computer-generated environment.[33]

Any VR system will consist of software, hardware, and input and output components.[34] Most VR environments are developed from images obtained in the real world, such as photographs or radiographic images. These images are converted using computer-aided design technology into computerized models consisting of large numbers of interlocking polygons that form the virtual image.[35] As with any computer program, increasing the quality of the image through increasing the number of polygons that form it results in a slower rate of update as the environment is navigated. This balance determines the level of realism that can be generated.[36] Advancing processor speeds have enabled progressively higher levels of fidelity over recent years, allowing complex VR simulation to be undertaken using commercially available computing technology.

In addition to the availability of relatively inexpensive VR technology, the delivery of VR simulation in medicine has advanced recently through the increasingly high-quality haptic technology. This technology offers both tactile and force feedback to the user, meaning that the sensation of passing through tissues of variable resistance can be mimicked in a real-time fashion. VR technology has been adopted most widely by surgeons and has shown benefits over conventional training alone in procedures such as colonoscopy; however, increasing interest has been shown in its use as both a procedural and investigation training tool in anesthesia and critical care.[37]

Procedural simulators for epidural insertion and fiberoptic bronchoscopy have been developed and offer insight into the potential uses of this kind of technology in anesthesia training.[38,39] Fiberoptic bronchoscopy and intubation of a VR simulator by pediatric trainees has been shown to result in a significantly reduced time to intubation in a real-life pediatric larynx.[39]

Considerable interest has been shown in the field of regional anesthesia in developing VR models to facilitate training in peripheral nerve blockade.[40] In a recent article, the problem of interindividual variability in regional anesthesia has been addressed in a series of patients undergoing MRI of their inguinal region, with that data used to create VR patients on whom trainees can practice.[41] In a further development, the combination of a traditional mannequin simulator with nonimmersive VR technology during resuscitation training has proven popular in an initial pilot.[42]

In terms of investigations, several tools have been developed using nonimmersive technology often combined with part-task simulators to offer trainees the ability to visualize the results of their actions and interact with the VR environment. An example of this is the HeartWorks echocardiography VR simulator developed by Inventive

Medical (University College London Hospitals, London, United Kingdom). The Heart-Works system offers the user the opportunity to undertake transesophageal echocardiography through manipulating a probe in the esophagus of a mannequin in real-time while visualizing the simulated ultrasound images alongside the corresponding sliced three-dimensional heart model.[43] There is also now a some evidence in the field of cardiothoracic anesthesia regarding the utility of TEE simulation devices in the training of novice anesthesia residents. The paper by Bose and colleagues[44] showed that this method was superior to traditional training in a number of clinically relevant areas.

COMPUTER/WEB-BASED SIMULATION TRAINING

Computer- and Internet-based simulation offers the simplest means of delivering simulation training to a large group of individuals. Although it lacks the level of interactivity of immersive simulators, the potential to engage in a wide range of situations through a readily available medium, such as the personal computer, has immediate appeal.

Most applications of computer-based simulations take the form of virtual patients. These virtual patients are used in either narrative or problem-solving exercises.[45,46] Problem-based learning is now much more widely used in medical training, particularly in medical student education.[47,48] It involves the participant garnering information from several sources to arrive at a management or diagnostic decision. In computer simulation, this is often delivered through drop-down menus offering information on patient history, examination findings, or test results. The goal is for the student to identify and pursue that correct choice without the need for external guidance. In a narrative process, the participant follows a predetermined course and is often required to show the importance of time or cause-and-effect relationships during a clinical situation.

The Internet has enabled broad access to computer-based simulations, with a reduced requirement for program installation, and although the limitations of remote access, particularly to large files, has been a problem in the past, the rapid improvement in download speeds has reduced these problems significantly.[49,50]

Advantages of this computer-based training include ease of access, the ability for facilities to accommodate multiple users simultaneously, and ease of monitoring of progress and performance.[51]

A large number of tools have been developed to exploit this technology. These instruments range from effective and popular programs designed to simulate responses to specific interventions, such as anesthetic gases and the pharmacokinetic responses to them, to complex problem-based learning packages, such as Web-SP, that offer students the facility to interact with all portions of a case, diagnose and manage problems, and receive structured feedback on their performance all without external involvement. Feedback from this kind of simulation has been strongly positive.[52,53]

Computer-based packages that have been developed for use in anesthesia and critical care include those with the ability to teach and assess participants on a series of resuscitation (ACLS Simulator, Anesoft, Issaquah, Washington) and critical care cases (Critical Care Simulator, Anesoft), including interpretation of clinical findings and tests, and knowledge of algorithms, ventilation, fluids, and drug dosages. These programs have been shown to be an inexpensive and popular method of training anesthesia residents, resulting in improved confidence in the management of emergency situations.[53] Training on a computer-based package before undertaking immersive simulation training has also been shown to result in improved performance in the simulations.[54] This finding may offer further evidence that integration of differing tools might offer an economically viable way to increase the productivity of simulation as a whole. In terms of assessment, computer-based tools have shown a degree of correlation with traditional knowledge assessments used in anesthesia training in the United States,[55] although they are not widely used as assessment tools, perhaps because of a lack of robust evidence for their use.

Other computer-only–based simulators available for use include MEDIQ Anaesthesia Simulator (MEDIQ Abraxas AB, Stockholm, Sweden) which is a desktop tool that can reproduce a series of complete operations with a high level of interactivity.[56] In addition, the University of Florida has developed the Virtual Anesthesia Machine, an online resource designed to show the function and modes of operation of different anesthetic machines.[57] The same group has also expanded their portfolio to include pharmacokinetic and difficult airway models.

An alternative approach is to used a computer-based simulation in conjunction with theater equipment to simulate observations, such as with the ACCESS package. This computer-driven simulation is relatively simple and inexpensive and is both well received and offers some evidence of construct validity in its ability to differentiate between experienced and novice anaesthetists.[58]

SUMMARY

Anesthesia has led the way in many areas of simulation training, with tools developed for use in immersive, VR, and computer-based training. It was recently suggested that a set of standards be introduced to guide the development of simulation in health care to achieve the full potential of this invaluable resource.[59]

The continued evolution of these tools depends on several factors. The availability of faculty who are skilled in the use of simulation equipment and also in structured feedback is essential; without this, the quality of training delivered will be impaired regardless of the available technology. With this comes the requirement for consistency in software and hardware design, along with high levels of usability to facilitate the uptake of these tools. Furthermore, willingness among practitioners to share their experience and learning resources will mean that the "simulation wheel" is not reinvented in multiple centers trying to achieve the same outcome.

The development of simulation training of any kind in a health care environment requires investment in equipment, facilities, and faculty development. The ongoing costs of equipment servicing and time away from clinical service provision for faculty and participants must also be taken into consideration. A cost/benefit relationship between simulation and clinical expenditure is difficult to show. In the current economic climate, education budgets and particularly simulation programs may suffer unless their funding is protected or a compelling case for their use can be made to those who allocate resources.

The future of simulation training in medicine might be divided into two phases: the completion of high-quality research and integration into the curriculum. The need to show value in medical education in terms of outcome-based measures is now widely accepted and simulation must conform to this process.[60] To achieve that, cooperation between institutions to generate studies of rigorous methodology and adequate sample size is essential. Additionally, further developments in technology in all branches of simulation will add to realism, reduce costs, and increase usability.

When adequate evidence becomes available, the next step will be to ensure that maximum value is achieved with the simulation tools available, which will require fully integrating equipment and skills into the educational curriculum of students, trainees, and specialists. A broad range of areas of training exist in which simulation might play a role. Focus must be placed on identifying the correct educational goals for the appropriate groups. For example, an emphasis on high-level leadership and nontechnical skills in doctors in their first postgraduate year might be less useful than putting the emphasis on the technical skills of initial assessment and management of the acutely unwell patient.

The sequential use of different simulation technologies to reduce costs and achieve maximum benefit is another area for exploration in the near future. The question is whether learners developing technical skills in central venous cannulation can use VR simulation to improve manual dexterity before integrating these skills into complete procedures during rehearsal in higher-fidelity environments.[61]

With the changes in medical training and working hours, the role of the doctor within the multidisciplinary team has become even more critical. The quality of work within these groups might be facilitated through interprofessional training in simulation centers and in local clinical environments using high-fidelity simulation to develop nontechnical skills among participants.[62]

Simulation in all its forms may well have a key role to play in medical education at all levels in the future. For now the focus must be on developing a robust body of evidence for its efficacy and ensuring that adequate resources are available to facilitate this use.

REFERENCES

1. Gorman PJ, Meier AH, Krummel TM. Simulation and virtual reality in surgical education: real or unreal? Arch Surg 1999;134:1203–8.
2. Issenberg S, McGachie W, Petrusa E, et al. Features and uses of high-fidelity medical simulations that lead to effective learning: a BEME (Best Evidence Medical Education) systematic review. Med Teach 2005;27:10–28.
3. Winchell SW, Safar P. Teaching lay and paramedical personnel in cardiopulmonary resuscitation. Anaesth Analg 1966;45:441–9.
4. Denson J, Abrahamson S. A computer controlled patient simulator. JAMA 1969; 208:504–8.
5. Gordon MS. Cardiology patient simulator: development of an automated mannekin to teach cardiovascular disease. Am J Cardiol 1974;34:350–5.
6. Woolliscroft JO, Calhoun JG, Tenhaken JD, et al. Harvey: the impact of a cardiovascular teaching simulator on student skill acquisition. Med Teach 1987;9:53–7.
7. Gordon MS, Ewy GA, Felner JM, et al. A cardiology patient simulator for continuing education of family physicians. J Fam Pract 1981;13:353–6.
8. Gordon MS, Eey GA, Felner JM, et al. Teaching bedside cardiologic skills using 'Harvey' the cardiology patient simulator. Med Clin North Am 1980;64:305–13.
9. Karnath BB, Thornton W, Frye AW. Teaching and testing physical examination skills without the use of patients. Acad Med 2002;77:753.
10. Gaba DM, DeAnda A. A comprehensive anaesthesia simulator environment: recreating the operating room for research and training. Anesthesiology 1988;69: 387–94.
11. Good M, Lam potang S, Gibby G, et al. Critical events simulation for training in anaesthesiology. J Clin Monit Comput 1988;4:140.
12. Good M, Grovenstein J, Mahjla M, et al. Can simulation accelerate learning of basic anesthesia skills by beginning residents? [abstract]. Anesthesiology 1992;77:A1133.
13. Chopra V, Engbers F, Geerts M, et al. The Leiden anaesthesia simulator. Br J Anaesth 1994;73:287–92.

14. Weinstock P, Kappus L, Kleinman M, et al. Toward a new paradigm in hospital-based pediatric education: The development of an onsite simulator program. Pediatr Crit Care Med 2005;6:635–41.
15. Hammam W. In-situ simulation: using aviation principles to identify relevant teamwork and systems issues to promote patient safety. Cambridge (MA): CRICO/RMF Forum; 2008.
16. Reason J. Managing the risk of organizational accidents. Brookfield (VT): Ashgate; 1997.
17. Herzer K, Rodriguez-Paz M, Doyle P, et al. A practical framework for patient care teams to prospectively identify and mitigate clinical hazards. Jt Comm J Qual Patient Saf 2009;35:72–81.
18. Wayne D, Didwania A, Feinglass J, et al. Simulation-based education improves quality of care during cardiac arrest team responses at an academic teaching hospital. Chest 2008;133:56–61.
19. Wayne D, Butter J, Siddall VJ, et al. Simulation-based training of internal medicine residents in advanced cardiac life support protocols: a randomized trial. Teach Learn Med 2005;17:210–6.
20. Wayne D, Siddall V, Butter J, et al. A longitudinal study of internal medicine residents' retention of advanced cardiac life support (ACLS) skills. Acad Med 2006; 81(Suppl):S9–12.
21. Rodriguez-Paz J, Mark L, Herzer K, et al. Using in-situ simulation to establish a new intraoperative therapy program: a novel multidisciplinary paradigm to patient safety [abstract: 53]. Presented at the International Meeting on Simulation in Healthcare. San Diego, January 15, 2008.
22. Kobayashi L, Patterson M, Overly F, et al. Educational and research implications of portable human patient simulation in acute care medicine. Acad Emerg Med 2008;15:1166–74.
23. Gaba DM. Improving anaesthesiologists performance by simulating reality. Anesthesiology 1992;76:491–4.
24. SimMan 3G Technical Specifications. Available at: http://www.laerdal.co.uk/doc/36969216/SimMan-3G.html#/specs. Accessed June 16, 2010.
25. Sevdalis N, Undre S, Henry J, et al. Development, initial reliability and validity testing of an observational tool for assessing technical skills of operating room nurses. Int J Nurs Stud 2009;46:1187–93.
26. Martin JA, Regehr G, Reznick R, et al. Objective structured assessment of technical skills (OSATS) for surgical residents. Br J Surg 1997;84:273–8.
27. Copper JB, Newbower RS, Kitz RJ. An analysis of major errors and equipment failures in anaesthesia management: considerations for prevention and detection. Anesthesiology 1984;60:34–42.
28. Helmrich R. On error management: lessons from aviation. BMJ 2000;320:781–5.
29. Helmreich RL, Merritt AC, Wilhelm JA. The evolution of crew resource management training in commercial aviation. Int J Aviat Psychol 1999;9:19–32.
30. Fletcher G, Flin R, McGeorge P, et al. Anaesthetists non technical skills (ANTS): evaluation of a behavioural marker system. Br J Anaesth 2003;90:580–8.
31. O'Conner P, Höermann H-J, Flin R, et al. Developing a method for evaluating crew resource management skills: a European perspective. Int J Aviat Psychol 2002; 12:263–85.
32. Fletcher G, McGeorge P, Flin R. The role of non technical skills in anaesthesia: a review of current literature. Br J Anaesth 2002;88:418–29.
33. Reznek M, Hartner P, Krummel T. Virtual reality and simulation: training the future emergency physician. Acad Emerg Med 2002;9:78–87.

34. Ahmed M, Meech JF, Timoney A. Virtual reality in medicine. Br J Urol 1997; 80(Suppl 3):45–62.
35. Burt DE. Virtual reality in anaesthesia. Br J Anaesth 1995;75:472–80.
36. Rawn CL, Gorman PJ, Graham WP, et al. Virtual reality becomes reality in plastic surgery. Perspect Plast Surg 2000;14:105–18.
37. Park J, MacRae H, Musselman L, et al. Randomised controlled trial of virtual reality simulator training: transfer to live patients. Am J Surg 2007;194:205–11.
38. Kneebone R. Simulation in surgical training: educational issues and practical training. Med Educ 2003;37:267–77.
39. Rowe R, Cohen RA. An evaluation of a virtual reality airway simulator. Anesth Analg 2002;95:62–6.
40. Ullrich S, Frommen T, Rossaint R, et al. Virtual reality-based regional anaesthesia simulator for axillary nerve blocks. Stud Health Technol Inform 2009;142:392–4.
41. Grottke O, Ntouba A, Ullrich S, et al. Virtual reality based simulator for training in regional anaesthesia. Br J Anaesth 2009;103:594–600.
42. Semeraro S, Frisoli A, Bergomasco M, et al. Virtual reality enhanced mannequin (VREM) that is well received by resuscitation experts. Resusc 2009;80:489–92.
43. Bose R, Matyal R, Panzica P, et al. Transesophageal echocardiography simulator: a new learning tool. J Cardiothorac Vasc Anesth 2009;23:544–8.
44. Bose RR, Matyal R, Warraich HJ, et al. Utility of a transesophageal echocardiographic simulator as a teaching tool. J Cardiothorac Vasc Anesth 2001;25:212–5.
45. Bearman M, Cesnik B, Liddell M. Randomised comparison of virtual patient models in the context of teaching clinical communication skills. Med Educ 2001;35:824–32.
46. Bearman M, Cesnik B. Comparing student attitudes to different models of the same virtual patient. Stud Health Technol Inform 2001;10:1004–8.
47. Narrows HS, Mitchell OM. An innovative course in undergraduate neuroscience. An experiment in problem-based learning with problem boxes. Br J Med Educ 1975;1(9):223–30.
48. Pales J, Gual A. Active and problem based learning: two years experience in physiology at medical school university of Barcelona. Med Educ 1992;26:442–72.
49. Haag M, Mayelin L, Tonshoff B, et al. Web based training: a new paradigm in computer assisted instruction in medicine. Int J Med Inf 1999;53:79–90.
50. Yamakawa T, Toyabe S, Cao P. Web-based delivery of medical multimedia contents using an MPEG-4 system. Comput Methods Programs Biomed 2004; 75:259–64.
51. Zary N, Johnson G, Boberg J, et al. Development, implementation and pilot evaluation of a web-based virtual patient case simulation environment—Web-SP. BMC Med Educ 2006;6:10.
52. Garfield JM, Paskin S, Philip JH. An evaluation of the effectiveness of a computer simulation of anaesthetic uptake and distribution as a teaching tool. Med Educ 1989;23:457–62.
53. Schwid HA, Souter K. Cost-effectiveness of screen-based simulation for anesthesiology residents: 18 year experience. American Society of Anesthesiologists Annual Meeting. New Orleans, LA, 2009.
54. Schwid HA, Rooke GA, Ross BK, et al. Anesoft anesthesia simulator improves performance in mannequin-based simulator: anesthesia Simulator improves performance in mannequin-based simulator. Teach Learn Med 2001;13:92–6.
55. Ludwig TA, Schwid HA. Use of the Anesoft anesthesia simulator to evaluate resident performance: preliminary validation of screen-based simulator for evaluating resident performance. Anesthesiology 2004;101:A1337.

56. MediQ Desktop Simulation Software. Available at: http://www.mediq.se/ansim4. htm. Accessed June 16, 2010.
57. Centre for safety, simulation and advanced learning technologies. Available at: http://vam.anest.ufl.edu/simulations/simulationportfolio.php. Accessed June 16, 2010.
58. Byrne A, Hilton P, Lunn J. Basic simulations for anaesthetists: a pilot study of the ACCESS system. Anaesthesia 1994;49:376–81.
59. Cumin D, Weller J, Henderson K, et al. Standards for simulation in anaesthesia: creating confidence in the tools. Br J Anaes 2010;105:45–51.
60. Morrison J. Outcomes based education for a changing health service. Med Educ 2005;39:648–9.
61. Kneebone R. Practice, rehearsal, and performance: an approach for simulation-based surgical and procedure training. JAMA 2009;302:1336–8.
62. Bradley P. The history of simulation in medical education and possible future directions. Med Educ 2006;40:254–62.

SECTION 3:
Bonus Articles

Edited by Alan D. Kaye, MD, PhD

Amiodarone Supplants Lidocaine in ACLS and CPR Protocols

Anna Mizzi, MD[a],*, Thanh Tran[b], Devanand Mangar, MD[b],
Enrico M. Camporesi, MD[c]

KEYWORDS

- Amiodarone • Ventricular tachyarrhythmias • Cardiac surgery
- ACLS protocol

Amiodarone is an antiarrhythmic medication used to treat and prevent certain types of serious, life-threatening ventricular arrhythmias. Amiodarone gained slow acceptance outside the specialized field of cardiac antiarrhythmic surgery because the side effects are significant. Recent adoption of amiodarone in the ACLS (Advanced Cardiac Life Support) protocol has somewhat popularized this class of antiarrhythmics. Its use is slowly expanding in the acute medicine setting of anesthetics. This article summarizes the use of amiodarone by anesthesiologists in the operating room and during cardio-pulmonary resuscitation (CPR).

SUDDEN CARDIAC DEATH

In a population of 1000, the average annual occurrence of sudden cardiac death (SCD) is approximately 0.2%, but population-related frequency of cardiovascular disease in different areas of the country should be considered. There are approximately 400,000 to 450,000 recorded occurrences of SCD in the United States, which accounts for about 60% of all cardiovascular mortality in this country.[1] Holter studies further indicate that approximately 85% percent of SCDs are caused by ventricular tachyarrhythmias, both pulseless ventricular tachycardia (VT) and ventricular fibrillation (VF).

VT is a critical condition that can lead to VF. VT is characterized as monomorphic when waveforms are at a steady rate and amplitude, and polymorphic when they are inconsistently variable. VF is another critical condition whereby the ventricles tremble rather than contract. VF waveforms are inconsistent in rate and amplitude,

[a] Department of Cardiothoracic and Vascular Anesthesia, San Raffaele Hospital, "Vita e Salute" University, Milan, Italy
[b] Florida Gulf-to-Bay Anesthesiology, 1 Tampa General Circle, Suite A327, Tampa, FL 33606, USA
[c] Department of Surgery/Anesthesiology, Florida Gulf-to-Bay Anesthesiology Associates & University of South Florida, 1 Tampa General Circle, Suite A327, Tampa, FL 33606, USA
* Corresponding author. 1 Tampa General Circle, Suite A327, Tampa, FL 33606.
E-mail address: anna.mizzi@alice.it

Anesthesiology Clin 29 (2011) 535–545
doi:10.1016/j.anclin.2011.05.001
1932-2275/11/$ – see front matter © 2011 Elsevier Inc. All rights reserved.
anesthesiology.theclinics.com

often more than 300 beats per minute and more than 0.2 mV in amplitude. The irregular rate and amplitude indicates the inconsistent and hectic electrical activity and contraction when the heart stops pumping. VF waveforms often weaken to asystole within 15 minutes.[2]

In countries with prosperous resources, such as the United States and Europe, cardiac arrest due to VT or VF is mostly caused by myocardial ischemia. As a consequence, major risk factors for SCD include those factors that can accelerate coronary artery disease. Other risk factors associated with SCD include age (typically 45–75 years), male sex, and dilated cardiomyopathy.[2]

Cardiac arrest due to VT or VF causes an interruption in oxygen supply that can lead to critical ischemic damage to the organs. This condition is life-threatening, and leads to death within minutes if untreated. The treatments for pulseless ventricular tachyarrhythmias include use of defibrillation and antiarrhythmic drugs.[3]

CARDIAC ACTION POTENTIALS

Cardiac action potentials are divided into fast-response action potential and slow-response action potential. Fast-response action potential, also known as nonpacemaker action potential, is found in nonnodal cardiomyocytes (atrial and ventricular myocytes, and Purkinje tissue). This action potential type relies on fast sodium channels for depolarization. Slow-response action potentials, on the other hand, also known as pacemaker action potentials, are found in nodal tissue, which consists of sinoatrial and atrioventricular nodes, and depend on calcium channels rather than sodium channels for depolarization (**Fig. 1**).[4]

Cardiac action potentials, in general, use sodium and calcium channels for depolarization, and potassium channels for repolarization. In fast-response action potential, phase 0 represents depolarization, whereby sodium channels open to enhance positive membrane potential. Phase 1 is the initial repolarization, when potassium channels open and allow outward K^+ current. There is, however, a slow increase in inward Ca^{2+} current during this time, impeding the repolarization seen in phase 2. This phase, however, lengthens the period of action potential, and is the only phase that shows a difference between cardiac action potentials and those of the nerves and skeletal muscle. Phase 3 is then the continuation of the repolarization, and phase 4 allows the action potential to return to resting membrane potential.[4]

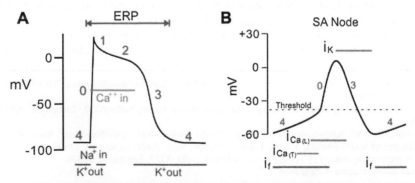

Fig. 1. Cardiac action potential. (*A*) Fast-response action potential (atrial and ventricular myocytes, and Purkinje tissue). (*B*) Slow-response action potential (sinoatrial and atrioventricular nodes). ERP, effective refractory period; SA, sinoatrial.

VAUGHAN WILLIAMS CLASSIFICATION

Antiarrhythmic drugs have different effects on action potentials, and are classified based on their mechanism of action. Many proposals have been made in classifying the antiarrhythmic drugs, but Vaughan Williams' classification seems to be the most used.[5] There are 4 classes in Vaughan Williams' classification, which are shown in **Table 1**.

Class I

Class I antiarrhythmics act as sodium channel blockers. These antiarrhythmics attach to and block sodium channels accountable for rapid depolarization in fast-response cardiac action potentials. The faster the depolarization of a cell, the faster adjacent cells would be depolarized, causing a faster regeneration and conduction of action potentials between the cells. Blocking sodium channels would decrease the action potential conduction velocity, and this action is helpful in repressing irregular conduction that can cause tachycardias.

Table 1	
Vaughan Williams classification for antiarrhythmic drugs	
CLASS I → Sodium Channel Blockers	
IA	• Moderate Na$^+$ channel blocking effect with conduction impairment • Prolonged repolarization • Quinide, Procainamide, Disopyramide
IB	• Minimal Na$^+$ channel blocking effect • Tendency for shortening repolarization • Lidocaine, Mexiletine, Tocainide
IC	• Marked Na$^+$ channel blocking effect with significant conduction impairment (QRS prolonged) • No effect on repolarization • Flecainide, Propafenone, Ethmozine
CLASS II → β-Receptor Antagonists	
• Depressed automaticity and conduction in slow-response cells • Impair calcium release to reduce contractility • No effect on repolarization • β-Blockers	
CLASS III → Potassium Channel Blockers	
• Potassium channel blockade lengthens refractoriness by delaying recovery of membrane potential • Most agents are not purely potassium blockers and have properties of other classes • Amiodarone, Bretylium, Azimilide, Dofetilide, Ibutilide	
CLASS IV	
IVA → Calcium channel blockers	• Predominantly blocks calcium entry in slow-response cells only (SA and AV nodal cells) • No effect on repolarization • Verapamil, Diltiazem
IVB → Adenosine receptor agonist	• Stimulation of adenosine receptor results in opening of potassium channels with predominant effect of hyperpolarization; This will depress automaticity in SA nodal cells and conduction in AV nodal cells • Minimal effect of shortening repolarization • Adenosine

Abbreviations: AV, atrioventricular; SA, sinoatrial.

Class I is further broken down to subclasses A, B, and C. These subclasses are based on the drugs' ability to alter action potential duration (APD) and effective refractory period (ERP). ERP is also known as absolute refractory period, and indicates the period in which, with an action potential already started, a new action potential cannot be started until the cell returns to resting membrane potential. Increasing or decreasing APD or ERP can increase or decrease arrhythmias based on the cause of the condition. Class IA increases APD and ERP, whereas class IB decreases APD and ERP, and IC has no effect on APD and ERP. Class IA drugs are classified as moderate sodium channel blockers, whereas IB drugs are weak and IC drugs are strong. Class IA drugs are used to treat atrial fibrillation, flutter, and supraventricular and ventricular tachyarrhythmias. Class IB drugs are used to treat ventricular tachyarrhythmias. Class IC drugs are used to treat life-threatening supraventricular and ventricular tachyarrhythmias.[6,7]

Class II

Class II drugs are known as β-blockers. β-Blockers attach to β-adrenoceptors in cardiac nodal tissue, the conducting system, and contracting myocytes to block catecholamines (noradrenaline and adrenaline) from binding to the adrenoceptors. β-Blockers are further divided into β1-blockers and β2-blockers. The heart has both β-adrenoceptors, but β1 predominate in number and function. β-Receptors bind norepinephrine released from sympathetic adrenergic nerves, as well as norepinephrine and epinephrine in the blood.

β-Blockers can reduce sympathetic influences that usually stimulate chronotropy (heart rate), inotropy (contractility), dromotropy (electrical conduction), and lusitropy (relaxation). Therefore, β-blockers would enable a reduction in heart rate, contractility, conduction velocity, and relaxation rate. β-Blockers are used to treat hypertension, angina, myocardial infarction, arrhythmias, and heart failure, and have been proposed as protective strategy to prevent perioperative cardiac events in patients undergoing major surgery.[8–10]

Class III

Class III drugs are known as potassium channel blockers and comprise amiodarone. Class III drugs bind and block the potassium channels used for repolarization, thus slowing down the repolarization process. By delaying repolarization, APD and effective ERP would increase. Drugs that help increase ERP are effective in suppressing tachyarrhythmias caused by reentry mechanisms. Potassium channel blockers are used to treat supraventricular and ventricular arrhythmias, life-threatening arrhythmias, and atrial fibrillation and flutter.[11–13]

Class IV

Class IV drugs are known as calcium channel blockers. These drugs bind to L-type calcium channels on vascular smooth muscle, cardiac myocytes, and cardiac nodal tissue. These channels regulate calcium entry into myocytes that stimulate smooth muscle and cardiac myocyte contractions. Calcium entry block enables calcium channel blockers to cause vasodilation, and decrease contractility, heart rate, and conduction velocity. Calcium channel blockers are administered for hypertension, angina, and arrhythmia therapies.[14–16]

LIDOCAINE, PROCAINAMIDE, AND BRETYLIUM

Procainamide and bretylium historically had an important clinical presence in ACLS and PALS (Pediatric Advanced Life Support), but today amiodarone is considered the drug of choice in cardiac arrest. Lidocaine continues to be an important drug, but is considered more as a local anesthetic than as an antiarrhythmic.

HISTORY OF AMIODARONE

Even though amiodarone was discovered in 1962, it was not put into use until 1967. Amiodarone was primarily used as an antianginal drug. In 1969, it was promoted to be used more specifically as an antiarrhythmic drug. The use of amiodarone as an antiarrhythmic to treat supraventricular and ventricular arrhythmias occurred primarily in France, South America, and the Scandinavian countries. By the mid-1980s, intravenous amiodarone was commonly used in Europe. In 1985, amiodarone gained approval by the US Food and Drug Administration (FDA). However, as harmful effects arose repeatedly, amiodarone was no longer viewed as an ideal antiarrhythmic.[17] By the mid-1990s, amiodarone was being used as "reserve antiarrhythmic" when other antiarrhythmic agents failed. By the start of the millennium, amiodarone regained its position as the ideal antiarrhythmic in treating VT and VF, as suggested in the ACLS algorithm.[18]

AMIODARONE AS AN ANTIARRHYTHMIC

Amiodarone, also known as Pacerone or Cordarone, is an antiarrhythmic agent that acts by reducing heart rate when it is too fast, such as in VF, tachycardia, atrial fibrillation, and atrial flutter. Amiodarone is categorized in Vaughan Williams Class III, where its properties include inhibiting potassium channels, protracting action potential duration and ERP, and averting recurring arrhythmias. Even though amiodarone is classified as Class III, it does also have effects seen in Class I, II, and IV; however, the main mechanism of action is not yet known.

Acute arrhythmias are usually treated with a pump-infusion system to deliver constant intravenous dose of amiodarone, whereas patients with chronic arrhythmias and children may receive an oral administration as amiodarone hydrochloride.

Amiodarone molecule composition consists of 37.3% iodine in weight (**Fig. 2**). Due to this iodine composition, amiodarone is known to cause many adverse effects concerning thyroidal complications when administered chronically.

Amiodarone can be advantageous in stabilizing monomorphic and polymorphic VT, and other tachycardias. Metabolism of amiodarone is rather intricate. Intravenously, amiodarone's half-life is short just as the distribution is large, and the redistribution goes to the fat, liver, heart, and brain. Redistribution is slow, approximately a few hours or days, while amiodarone stays in the serum for about 12 to 24 hours. As

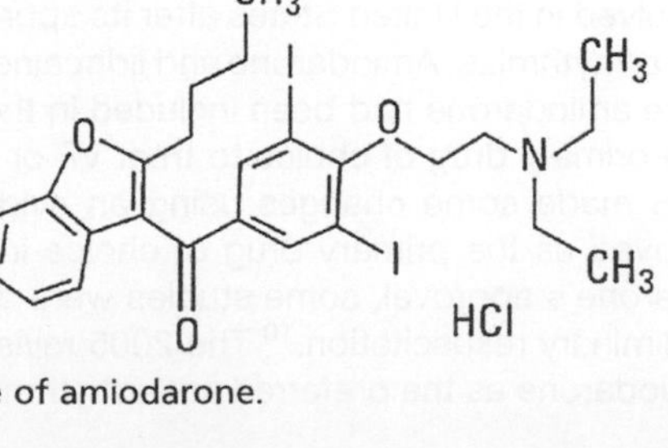

Fig. 2. Chemical structure of amiodarone.

amiodarone is metabolized via the liver, it evolves to become desethylamiodarone, a Vaughan Williams Class III antiarrhythmic.[19–22]

ADVERSE EFFECTS OF AMIODARONE

Amiodarone has numerous side effects. Most individuals administered amiodarone on a chronic basis will experience at least one side effect.

The most serious reaction caused by amiodarone is interstitial lung disease. Risk factors include high cumulative dose, more than 400 mg per day, duration over 2 months, age, and preexisting pulmonary disease. Common practice is to avoid using the agent if possible in individuals with decreased lung function. The most specific test of pulmonary toxicity due to amiodarone is a dramatic reduction in gas exchange, measurable by a decreased diffusion capacity of carbon monoxide on pulmonary function testing.[23]

Thyroxine and amiodarone have similar structures. Due to the iodine content of the agent, abnormalities in thyroid function are common. Both underactivity and overactivity of the thyroid may occur while on amiodarone treatment. Measurement of free thyroxine (FT_4) alone may be unreliable in detecting these problems, so thyroid-stimulating hormone (TSH) should also be checked every 6 months.[23–25]

Corneal microdeposits (corneal verticillata, also called vortex keratopathy) are almost universally present (>90%) in individuals taking amiodarone for at least 6 months. These deposits typically do not cause any symptoms. Optic neuropathy occurs in 1% to 2% of people and is not dose dependent. Bilateral optic disk swelling and mild and reversible visual field defects can also occur.[26]

Long-term administration of amiodarone is associated with a blue-gray discoloration of the skin, more commonly seen in individuals with lighter skin tones. The discoloration may revert on cessation of the drug. However, the skin color may not return completely to normal.[27]

The most common adverse effect of intravenous amiodarone is hypotension.[28] This complication may possibly be associated with the infusion rate. Hypotension can be treated with vasopressor drugs, positive inotropic agents, and volume expansion therapies, or reduction of the infusion rate.

While amiodarone is known for its tachycardia treatments, it has proarrhythmic effects as well, such as bradycardia, asystole, and torsade de pointes. However, in clinical practice it might be difficult to differentiate between an insufficient dose of amiodarone and actual proarrhythmic effects. If the arrhythmias persist even with a higher dose and the patient is hemodynamically unstable, the drug should be ceased as soon as possible. QT interval analysis can help in reaching this decision. The problem is quite complex, as amiodarone can increase the QT interval while not inducing torsade de pointes, and can cause polymorphic VT while not stretching the QT interval.

AMIODARONE IN THE ACLS

Before its popularity evolved in the United States after its approval from the FDA, lidocaine was used to treat arrhythmias. Amiodarone and lidocaine are often used for CPR in cardiac arrest. Before amiodarone had been included in the ACLS algorithm, lidocaine was listed as the primary drug of choice to treat VF or VT (VF/VT). In 2000, as the guidelines in ACLS made some changes using an evidence-based approach, amiodarone was approved as the primary drug of choice in the ACLS tachycardia algorithm. After amiodarone's approval, some studies were also performed showing its effectiveness in preliminary resuscitation.[10] The 2005 revision of the ACLS guidelines also mentions amiodarone as the preferred antiarrhythmic drug of choice based on trials. ACLS guidelines now indicate that amiodarone must be the first antiar-rhythmic administered to treat VF/VT; and only after attempts at using amiodarone are ineffective can lidocaine and procainamide be used.[3]

TRIALS REGARDING AMIODARONE IN SUSTAINED VENTRICULAR TACHYARRHYTHMIAS AND CARDIAC ARREST

Even though lidocaine had been used to treat VF/VT for many years, there was lack of evidence for its usefulness over other drugs. Compared with other antiarrhythmics, more controlled data can be found for amiodarone. Based on comparison trials wherein it was tested with other antiarrhythmics, amiodarone has been shown to enhance survival to hospital admission; however, a benefit in survival to hospital discharge has not yet been found.[29–32]

Levine and colleagues[29] investigated the response to intravenous amiodarone in a prospective, double-blinded, randomized study of 273 patients with life-threatening ventricular arrhythmias causing systolic blood pressure to decrease to below 80 mm Hg with clinical signs and symptoms of shock. All patients included were refractory to lidocaine, procainamide, and bretylium, and were randomized to receive 1 of 3 doses of amiodarone: 525, 1050, or 2100 mg over 24 hours. The primary end point was to determine the proportion of patients who survived with no further episodes of hemodynamically instable VT. Secondary end points were survival during the first 24 hours, successful therapy, additional boluses of intravenous amiodarone, and proarrhythmic effect.

Of the 273 included patients, 110 (40%) survived within 24 hours without hypoten-sive ventricular tachyarrhythmia with amiodarone as a single antiarrhythmic. The number of supplemental doses of intravenous amiodarone was significantly greater in the 525-mg group than in the 2100-mg group ($P = .0043$). However, there was no clear dose-response correlation observed with respect to successful rate or mortality. This study concluded that amiodarone is a relatively safe therapy for hypotensive ventricular tachyarrhythmias.

In another randomized, double-blinded study,[30] amiodarone was compared with a placebo, polysorbate 80, a diluent for amiodarone, in 504 adults with nontrau-matic prehospital cardiac arrest with VF or pulseless VT who had not been resus-citated after 3 precordial shocks. Of these patients, 246 were randomized to receive 300 mg of intravenous amiodarone (only a single dose) while 258 received placebo. The primary end point was admission to the hospital with a spontaneously perfusing rhythm. Secondary end points were adverse effects, the number of pre-cordial shocks required after the study drug, the total duration of CPR, and the need for additional drugs. Eighty-eight percent of the patients had VF and 7% had pulseless VT. There was no significant difference between the two groups in the mean duration of the resuscitative efforts, the number of shocks, or the proportion of patients requiring additional antiarrhythmics. More patients receiving amiodarone had hypotension (59% vs 48%, $P = .04$) or bradycardia (41% vs 25%, $P = .004$). The patients in the amiodarone group were more likely to survive to be admitted to the hospital (44% vs 34%, $P = .03$). This trial showed that the administration of amiodarone resulted in a higher rate of survival to hospital admission in patients with prehospital cardiac arrest due to refractory ventricular tachyarrhythmias.

Another study[31] compared amiodarone and lidocaine in adult patients with preho-spital VF, resistant to 3 shocks, intravenous epinephrine, and a further shock. In total 347 patients were enrolled; 180 were randomized to receive amiodarone (5 mg/kg estimated body weight) while 167 received lidocaine (1.5 mg/kg). The primary end point was survival to admission to the hospital. Secondary end points included survival to discharge from the hospital and adverse events. After treatment with amiodarone, 22.8% of patients survived to hospital admission, as compared with 12.0% of patients treated with lidocaine ($P = .009$). Among the 41 patients who survived to hospital admission after receiving amiodarone, 9 survived to hospital discharge (5% of the entire group), as compared with 5 of the 20 initial survivors in the lidocaine group (3% of the entire group) ($P = .34$). The investigators concluded that if an antiarrhythmic drug is to be considered in patients with shock-resistant VF, intravenous amiodarone should be the drug of choice, due to higher rates of survival to hospital admission in patients receiving amiodarone as compared with lidocaine.

Pollak and colleagues[32] conducted a retrospective study in which charts of 347 patients who underwent cardiac resuscitation were studied to determine whether the use of amiodarone improved survival in the case of in-hospital cardiac arrest. The end points were survival of resuscitation effort to return of spontaneous circulation, and survival to discharge.

Pulseless VT or VF were present in 95 patients. Clinical uptake of amiodarone was limited; only 36 patients received amiodarone while 59 patients received other antiarrhythmics. In the 36 patients receiving amiodarone, survival of resuscitation was 67% vs 83% in the 59 patients receiving other drugs. Survival to discharge was 36.1% and 55.9% in the two groups, respectively. This study concluded that use of amiodarone was less than 50% and that no clinically observable survival benefit could be documented in in-hospital cardiac arrest. Possible explanations for the difference between this experience and that found in out-of-hospital resuscitation trials include differing patient populations and operator bias during resuscitation.

AMIODARONE IN CARDIAC SURGERY

Atrial fibrillation (AF) is an important and frequent complication after cardiac surgery, occurring in almost one-third of patients undergoing coronary artery bypass grafting and in up to 44% of patients undergoing a valvular procedure. Heart failure, hypotension, increased risk of stroke, need for anticoagulation, increased length of stay in the hospital, and long-term mortality are some of the various potential consequences of postoperative AF.

Postoperative AF was found to be significantly reduced in a double-blinded study[33] in which 124 patients were randomized to receive either oral amiodarone (64 patients) or placebo (60 patients) for a minimum of 7 days before elective cardiac surgery with cardiopulmonary bypass. Amiodarone dose was 600 mg/d for 7 days, then 200 mg/d until discharge from the hospital. The incidence of postoperative AF was 25% (16 patients) in the amiodarone group and 53% (25 patients) in the group receiving placebo ($P = .003$). Patients in the amiodarone group were hospitalized for significantly fewer days than those in placebo group (6.5 ± 2.6 vs 7.9 ± 4.3 days, $P = .04$), and total hospitalization costs were also significantly less in the amiodarone group ($P = .03$). No difference was found in the occurrence of postoperative complications between the two groups.

The safety of short-term amiodarone therapy with fentanyl-containing anesthesia was investigated in a randomized, double-blinded, placebo-controlled trial of cardiac surgical patients with fentanyl-isoflurane anesthesia.[34] There were 84 patients enrolled: 45 patients received amiodarone (3.4 g over 5 days or 2.2 g over 24 hours) while 39 received placebo. The primary end point was to compare the incidence of hemodynamic instability, defined as: net increase in fluid balance during surgery of more than 2 L, use of more than10 mg/kg/min dopamine, other vasopressive catecholamines, and need for a phosphodiesterase inhibitor or intra-aortic balloon pump. There were no significant differences between the two groups in any indicator for hemodynamic instability.

Although valvular surgery poses a greater risk for AF, most studies in cardiac surgery have been performed in patients undergoing coronary revascularization. In several of these protocols, the preoperative loading regimen was administered orally; however, this approach is currently impractical because most patients undergoing elective cardiac surgery are admitted the night before the procedure. Beaulieu and colleagues[35] randomized 120 patients to receive either amiodarone (intravenous loading dose after the induction of anesthesia followed by a 2-day perfusion) or placebo to compare the occurrence of postoperative AF. Postoperative AF occurred more frequently in patients who received amiodarone (59.3% vs 40.0% in the control group, $P = .035$). Four preoperative factors were found to be associated with a higher risk of postoperative AF: older age ($P = .0003$), recent myocardial infarction ($P = .026$), preoperative angina ($P = .0326$), and use of calcium channel blockers ($P = .0078$). This study showed that intravenous amiodarone administered in the perioperative period did not reduce the burden of postoperative AF in valvular surgery.

Amiodarone use during anesthesia for noncardiac procedures has not been described specifically, if not for patients requiring continuous antiarrhythmic therapy.

SUMMARY

Amiodarone is an antiarrhythmic drug that is useful to treat AF and perioperative tachyarrhythmias in cardiac surgery, and is the drug of choice for the treatment of out-of-hospital cardiac arrest as indicated in the ACLS protocol. Despite the promising results obtained in these settings, data about the use of amiodarone in noncardiac procedures are still lacking, and further studies are necessary to assess whether amiodarone can be advantageous.

REFERENCES

1. Rosamond W, Flegal K, Furie K, et al. Heart disease and stroke statistics—2008 update: a report from the American Heart Association Statistics Committee and Stroke Statistics Subcommittee. Circulation 2008;117:25–146.
2. Lang E, Al Raisi M. Ventricular tachyarrhythmias (out of hospital cardiac arrests). Clin Evid 2006;15:295–300.
3. International Liaison Committee on Resuscitation. 2005 International Consensus on cardiopulmonary resuscitation and emergency cardiovascular care science with treatment recommendations. Part 4: advanced life support. Resuscitation 2005;67(2/3):213–47. Available at: http://www.cvphysiology.com/index.html. Accessed May 21, 2011.
4. Klabunde R. Cardiovascular physiology concepts. Lippincott Williams & Wilkins; 2005.
5. Vaughan Williams EM. A classification of actions reassessed after a decade of new drugs. J Cardiovasc Pharmacol 1984;24:129–47.
6. Pallandi RT, Campbell TJ. Selective depression of conduction of premature action potentials in canine Purkinje fibres by class Ib antiarrhythmic drugs: comparison with Ia and Ic drugs. Cardiovasc Res 1988;22(3):171–8.
7. Man RY, Bril A. Effects of class I anti-arrhythmic drugs in infarcted tissue. Clin Invest Med 1991;14(5):466–75.

8. Zicha S, Tsuji Y, Shiroshita-Takeshita A, et al. Beta-blockers as antiarrhythmic agents. Handb Exp Pharmacol 2006;171:235–66.

9. Dorian P. Antiarrhythmic action of beta-blockers: potential mechanisms. J Cardiovasc Pharmacol Ther 2005;10(Suppl 1):S15–22.

10. Fleisher LA, Beckman JA, Brown KA, et al, American College of Cardiology Foundation/American Heart Association. Task Force on Practice Guidelines; American Society of Echocardiography; American Society of Nuclear Cardiology; Heart Rhythm Society; Society of Cardiovascular Anesthesiologists; Society for Cardiovascular Angiography and Interventions; Society for Vascular Medicine; Society for Vascular Surgery. ACCF/AHA focused update on perioperative beta blockade incorporated into the ACC/AHA 2007 guidelines on perioperative cardiovascular evaluation and care for noncardiac surgery. J Am Coll Cardiol 2009;54(22):e13–118.

11. Nattel S, Singh BN. Evolution, mechanisms, and classification of antiarrhythmic drugs: focus on class III actions. Am J Cardiol 1999;84(9A):11R–9R.

12. Khan MH. Oral class III antiarrhythmics: what is new? Curr Opin Cardiol 2004; 19(1):47–51.

13. Woosley RL, Funck-Brentano C. Overview of the clinical pharmacology of antiarrhythmic drugs. Am J Cardiol 1988;61(2):61A–9A.

14. Weir MR. Calcium channel blockers: their pharmacologic and therapeutic role in hypertension. Am J Cardiovasc Drugs 2007;7(Suppl 1):5–15.

15. Holdgate A, Foo A. Adenosine versus intravenous calcium channel antagonists for the treatment of supraventricular tachycardia in adults. Cochrane Database Syst Rev 2006;4:CD005154.

16. Sica DA. Pharmacotherapy review: calcium channel blockers. J Clin Hypertens (Greenwich) 2006;8(1):53–6.

17. Singh BN, Venkatesh N, Nademanee K, et al. The historical development, cellular electrophysiology and pharmacology of amiodarone. Prog Cardiovasc Dis 1989; 31(4):249–80.

18. de Latorre F, Nolan J, Robertson C, et al, European Resuscitation Council. European Resuscitation Council Guidelines 2000 for Adult Advanced Life Support. A statement from the Advanced Life Support Working Group(1) and approved by the Executive Committee of the European Resuscitation Council. Resuscitation 2001;48(3):211–21.

19. Ornato J. Cardiopulmonary resuscitation. Totowa (NJ): Humana Press Inc; 2005.

20. Zimetbaum P. Amiodarone for atrial fibrillation. N Engl J Med 2007;356:935–41.

21. London B. Amiodarone and atrial fibrillation. J Cardiovasc Electrophysiol 2007; 18(12):1321–2.

22. Lafuente-Lafuente C, Alvarez JC, Leenhardt A, et al. Amiodarone concentrations in plasma and fat tissue during chronic treatment and related toxicity. Br J Clin Pharmacol 2009;67(5):511–9.

23. Vorperian VR, Havighurst TC, Miller S, et al. Adverse effects of low dose amiodarone: a meta-analysis. J Am Coll Cardiol 1997;30(3):791–8.

24. Eskes SA, Wiersinga WM. Amiodarone and thyroid. Best Pract Res Clin Endocrinol Metab 2009;23(6):735–51.

25. Cohen-Lehman J, Dahl P, Danzi S, et al. Effects of amiodarone therapy on thyroid function. Nat Rev Endocrinol 2010;6(1):34–41.

26. Greene HL, Graham EL, Werner JA, et al. Toxic and therapeutic effects of amiodarone in the treatment of cardiac arrhythmias. J Am Coll Cardiol 1983;2(6):1114–28.

27. Reid L, Khammo N, Clothier RH. An evaluation of the effects of photoactivation of bithionol, amiodarone and chlorpromazine on human keratinocytes in vitro. Altern Lab Anim 2007;35(5):471–85.

28. Aranki SF, Shaw DP, Adams DH, et al. Predictors of atrial fibrillation after coronary artery surgery. Current trends and impact on hospital resources. Circulation 1996;94(3):390–7.
29. Levine JH, Massumi A, Scheinman MM, et al. Intravenous Amiodarone Multicenter Trial Group. Intravenous amiodarone for recurrent sustained hypotensive ventricular tachyarrhythmias. J Am Coll Cardiol 1996;27(1):67–75.
30. Kudenchuk PJ, Cobb LA, Copass MK, et al. Amiodarone for resuscitation after out-of-hospital cardiac arrest due to ventricular fibrillation. N Engl J Med 1999; 341(12):871–8.
31. Dorian P, Cass D, Schwartz B, et al. Amiodarone as compared with lidocaine for shock-resistant ventricular fibrillation. N Engl J Med 2002;346(12):884–90.
32. Pollak PT, Wee V, Al-Hazmi A, et al. The use of amiodarone for in-hospital cardiac arrest at two tertiary care centres. Can J Cardiol 2006;22(3):199–202.
33. Daoud EG, Strickberger SA, Man KC, et al. Preoperative amiodarone as prophylaxis against atrial fibrillation after heart surgery. N Engl J Med 1997;337(25): 1785–91.
34. White CM, Dunn A, Tsikouris J, et al. An assessment of the safety of short-term amiodarone therapy in cardiac surgical patients with fentanyl-isoflurane anesthesia. Anesth Analg 1999;89(3):585–9.
35. Beaulieu Y, Denault AY, Couture P, et al. Perioperative intravenous amiodarone does not reduce the burden of atrial fibrillation in patients undergoing cardiac valvular surgery. Anesthesiology 2010;112(1):128–37.

Voluven, A New Colloid Solution

Anna Mizzi, MD[a], Thanh Tran[b], Rachel Karlnoski, PhD[b,c,*],
Ashley Anderson, BS[b], Devanand Mangar, MD[b],
Enrico M. Camporesi, MD[b,d,e]

KEYWORDS

• Hydroxyethyl starch • Voluven • Colloids • Crystalloids

A variety of fluid solutions can be used as intravascular replacement for surgical volume loss, and to avoid or delay blood transfusions. Crystalloid solutions, such as Ringer lactate, are typically administered at a rate of 3 or 4 times the volume of blood loss caused by continuous rapid extravasations. Approximately 20% of the volume initially administered remains in the intravascular space hours later. Therefore, rapid infusion of large amounts of crystalloid solutions can cause problems in elderly patients with limited cardiovascular reserve, and can lead to pulmonary and systemic edema. Alternatively, a commonly used synthetic colloid, hydroxyethyl starch (HES), readily allows for a 1:1 replacement ratio of intravascular volume to shed blood, and remains in the intravascular space longer compared with crystalloid solutions. However, HES can induce coagulopathy during prolonged surgical procedures because of the reduced release of factor VIII, von Willebrand Factor (vWF), and impaired platelet function.

There are many types of HES according to molecular weight (MW) and degree of substitution (DS). In general, HES with a low MW and low DS is preferred because HES solutions with a high MW and high DS are harder to metabolize and eliminate from the intravascular space. This prolonged stay results in extended adverse effects on coagulation. Six percent HES with a MW of 130 kDa and a DS of 0.4 in a saline medium (Voluven, Fresenius Kabi, Germany) has the lowest MW/DS ratio among other HES on the market and therefore is purported to induce less coagulation impairment. This review of crystalloid and colloid fluid replacement alternatives explores recently published evidence of the clinical utility of Voluven.

---

[a] Department of Cardiothoracic and Vascular Anesthesia, San Raffaele Hospital, "Vita e Salute" University, Milan, Italy
[b] Florida Gulf-to-Bay Anesthesiology Associates, 1 Tampa General Circle Suite A327, Tampa, FL 33606, USA
[c] Department of Plastic Surgery, University of South Florida, Tampa, FL, USA
[d] Department of Surgery, University of South Florida, Tampa, FL, USA
[e] Department of Anesthesiology, University of South Florida, Tampa, FL, USA
* Corresponding author. Florida Gulf-to-Bay Anesthesiology Associates, 1 Tampa General Circle Suite A327, Tampa, FL 33606.
E-mail address: rkarlnoski@fgtba.com

Anesthesiology Clin 29 (2011) 547–555
doi:10.1016/j.anclin.2011.05.012   anesthesiology.theclinics.com

FLUID REPLACEMENT

Use of fluid replacement to retain bodily fluid balance requires knowledge of water, sodium, and colloid distribution in the body. Total body water includes approximately 28 L of intracellular fluid and 14 L of extracellular fluid. Plasma volume comprises approximately 3 L; and red blood cell volume comprises 2 L. The body as a whole depends on maintaining this balance in total body water. Therefore, efficient usage of fluid replacement with surgical blood loss is critical.

Blood transfusions offer the advantages of increased tissue oxygenation and reduced bleeding, but there are also associated risks, such as allergic reactions and infection. Although blood transfusions are beneficial, this method is costly and not always readily available. Another effective method in responding to surgical blood loss is the injection of crystalloid and/or colloid solutions to increase the intravascular volume rather than adding the amount lost directly.[1,2] Perioperative physiologic alterations and anesthesia can also lead to changes in fluid balance. Anesthesiologists must be able to respond and manage the balance, corresponding to fluid therapy.

COLLOIDS VERSUS CRYSTALLOIDS

Colloids and crystalloids are classifications of substances based on their diffusion rates through capillary membranes. In 1861, a study was performed by Thomas Graham observing different substances and classifying them into 2 categories of colloids and crystalloids based on their abilities to diffuse through parchment paper, which acted as a capillary membrane.[3] Substances that passed through the parchment paper readily were classified as crystalloids, whereas substances that passed through slowly were classified as colloids. Even today, the distinction between colloids and crystalloids is not completely clear for a specific substance because the phase can change in different conditions; for example, soap in water is considered a colloid, whereas soap submerged in alcohol is a crystalloid. However, the original hypothesis regarding the different capabilities when passing through a membrane still holds. Therefore, intravenous fluids are distinguished based on their abilities to diffuse through the capillary membrane and to distribute properly between the intravascular and extravascular spaces.[4]

In fluid therapy, there is much debate about the effectiveness of colloid versus crystalloid solutions. Colloid advocates argue that use of crystalloid solution attenuates the plasma oncotic pressure leading to fluid movement from the intravascular space to the interstitial space.[5] On the other hand, crystalloid advocates suggest that albumin molecules penetrate easily into the pulmonary interstitial space and exit through the lymphatic system returning to systemic circulation.[2]

CRYSTALLOIDS

Crystalloid fluids are often composed of salt solutions such as sodium chloride; therefore, they are inexpensive and readily accessible. These solutions are classified as isotonic, hypertonic, or hypotonic. As crystalloids consist of salts, their ions are small and capable of moving freely across the semipermeable capillary membrane. As a result of this free movement, crystalloid fluids tend to distribute evenly throughout the intravascular and extravascular space. This increases the interstitial volume rather than the plasma volume, which is the main component of extravascular fluid.[1] The required replacement of crystalloid is threefold or fourfold of the lost blood volume. The distribution of crystalloid is 1:4, meaning 3 L intravascularly and 12 L extravascularly. This distribution also indicates that the crystalloid would likely expand more in the extravascular space rather than the intravascular space.[2] Thus, injecting crystalloid fluids would likely result in expansion of the interstitial volume. As a consequence, large amounts need to be injected for the crystalloid fluids to remain in the intravascular space, increasing the plasma volume.[4]

Examples of Crystalloids

Some of the common crystalloids include normal or isotonic saline, lactated Ringer solution, Normosol or PlasmaLyte, hypertonic salt solutions, and dextrose.

Normal saline is a 0.9% sodium chloride solution. Because its chloride content is higher than that of plasma, hyperchloremic metabolic acidosis may occur.[4] Normal saline has no buffer or other electrolytes, and can be administered in patients with renal dysfunction because it contains no potassium.[2]

Lactated Ringer solution consists of potassium and calcium in a sodium chloride diluent. British physician Sydney Ringer's initial solution was developed in 1880 to induce heart contractions in frogs. Later, American pediatrician Alexis Hartmann proposed adding sodium to the solution to treat metabolic acidosis in the 1930s.[6] From then on the solution became popular in intravenous therapy. Because of the calcium content, lactated Ringer solution is not likely to be mixed with blood transfusions as the calcium binds to certain drugs, making them less effective (specifically anticoagulants). Lactated Ringer solution has not been seen to have any advantage over normal saline.[6]

Normosol or PlasmaLyte has the advantage of a buffer capacity making its pH equal to the pH of plasma. It is also advantageous in patients who show reduction in magnesium. However, this could be a disadvantage in patients with renal deficiency, inducing hypermagnesemia, when the kidney fails to excrete magnesium leading to high levels retained in the blood.[4]

Hypertonic salt solutions have concentrations ranging from 250 to 1200 mEq/L. Their required volumes are less than those of the other solutions due to greater sodium concentration. The reduced water injection, due to the osmotic pressure forcing water from the intracellular to extracellular space, may lead to edema reduction. Another major advantage of hypertonic saline is its effectiveness in field triage with trauma as it is inexpensive, easily stored, and capable of expanding the plasma volume quickly.[2] However, they are used less frequently than the other solutions.

Dextrose is often added to intravenous solutions to enhance osmolarity. When added to Ringer solution or normal saline, dextrose generates hypertonic infusion. Because dextrose is glucose, administering dextrose could cause cell dehydration in patients with glucose impairment. On the other hand, a useful adjunct of glucose infusion is suppression of muscle protein catabolism as suggested by Mikura and colleagues.[7]

COLLOIDS

Colloids are composed of large molecules, such as proteins, that cannot pass through a semipermeable membrane. Therefore, the solute concentration inside the cell is higher than that outside the cell, increasing the flow of water into the cell, thus building up a pressure called the oncotic pressure or colloid osmotic pressure. This oncotic pressure leads to an increase in volume of the intravascular section, specifically the plasma volume, rather than the interstitial space of the extravascular section. As a result, lesser amounts need to be injected for the colloid fluids to stay in the intravascular section compared with crystalloid fluids. The capability of each colloid solution to expand the volume of plasma is proportional to the oncotic pressure. When the oncotic pressure of the colloid solution exceeds the oncotic pressure of plasma, the expansion exceeds the volume of infusion. Colloid solutions, however, are more expensive than crystalloid solutions due to their content, such as protein extracted from the body.[1] Another advantage of colloids is that there is minimal to no risk of infection or transmission of viral diseases.[2]

Examples of Colloids

Colloids that are often used include different percentages of albumin, hetastarch, pentastarch, and dextran.[1]

Albumin is a blood-derived, transport protein that is prepared by heating methods, and is available as albumin 5% and 25% in normal saline diluent. Albumin at 25% is given in smaller volumes compared with 5% albumin because the amount of associated sodium is less. The oncotic pressure of 25% albumin is greater than the oncotic pressure of 5% albumin at 70 mmHg and 20 mmHg, respectively. Therefore, 25% albumin expands plasma volume more than 5% albumin. For example, when 100 mL of 25% albumin is infused, the plasma volume is said to expand to 400 to 500 mL. Heat-treated albumin eliminates any associated viral transmission, such as human immunodeficiency virus, which makes the patient more susceptible to infections.[4,8]

Hetastarch is commonly prepared as a 6% solution in normal saline. Hetastarch consists of amylopectin molecules, one of the constituents of starch. Amylopectin molecules are glucose polymers in plants that range in size from 100 to 1,000,000 Da. Hetastarch is a synthetic colloid that has a similar MW and effect to 5% albumin; but it is lower in cost and stronger because its higher oncotic pressure allows it to expand the plasma volume to 30 mmHg versus 20 mmHg with 5% albumin. To be excreted by kidneys, hetastarch molecules must first be cleaved by amylase enzymes, which can lead to an increase in amylase levels. These colloids can also affect the coagulation cascade; hetastarch can produce dilutional results like other volume expanders and decrease factor VIII and vWF levels. Hetastarch can also reduce the accessibility of glycoprotein IIb/IIIa on the surface of platelets.[9] All these effects on coagulation parameters can result in severe coagulopathy.

Pentastarch is a form of hetastarch that is lower in MW and consists of smaller molecules. As pentastarch has higher quantity and smaller molecules than hetastarch, it results in higher oncotic pressure and better expansion. Pentastarch is prepared as 10% in normal saline. It is often preferred over hetastarch because it is less likely to lead to the same undesirable effects, such as coagulopathy.[2] Pentastarch is mainly used in Europe, not the United States.

Dextrans are polymers of glucose from the bacterium *Leuconostoc*, developed in a medium made up of sucrose. Dextrans are available as 10% dextrans 70 and 40 in normal saline. Dextran 70 is a volume expander, whereas dextran 40 is used to increase blood flow. Both dextrans have an oncotic pressure of 40 mmHg, greater than that of plasma at 20 mmHg. Dextran 40 is a better short-term volume expander than dextran 70, particularly for a few hours compared with the lengthened effect of dextran 70. Thus, dextran 70 is often preferred over dextran 40. Dextran can be antigenic and can lead to anaphylactoid reactions, but the incidence of such severe reactions has been reduced dramatically from about 5% to 0.032% in the past 20 years. Dextrans can disable the crossmatch for blood by coating red blood cells and increasing the erythrocyte sedimentation rate. Dextrans are also considered as a cause of acute renal failure because their oncotic pressure is higher than plasma, reducing filtration pressure in the kidneys.[2,10]

HES 130/0.4 (Voluven, Fresenius/Hospira, Germany): A New Colloid

HES is derived from amylopectin, a polysaccharide from maize, and is similar to glycogen. HES is prepared by hydrolysis, in vivo, by serum α-amylase and amylopectin hydroxyethylation. Hydroxyethylation, which is also known as molar substitution, helps to identify the different starches. Hydroxyethyl substitution causes the solubility of starch to increase and delays hydrolysis, thus delaying the degradation of starch molecules and excretion.[11]

HES is excreted by the kidneys and the rate of decomposition of starch is based on the molar substitution and C2/C6 ratio, which is the substitution of hydroxyethyl at the C2 or C6 location. The higher the molar substitution and C2/C6 ratios, the slower the decomposition, ultimately leading to plasma accumulation. The higher molar substitution means a larger molecule; so the larger the molecule, the slower the degradation in the body.[12]

Another form of starch that is now in favor as an alternative to older HES is Voluven. The United States Food and Drug Administration approved the use of Voluven for intravenous treatment of blood loss in December 2007.[13] **Table 1** compares Voluven pharmacokinetics with hetastarch (Hespan, B. Braun Medical) and albumin. Voluven, like hetastarch and pentastarch, consists of artificial starch that is insoluble in water. Voluven is also mixed in a salt solution so that its salt concentration is similar to that in blood. Also like the older starches, this newly introduced starch acts as a plasma volume expander.[11]

The average MW of Voluven is 130,000 Da. The ratio of hydroxyethyl group substitution to the glucose units, or molar substitution, in the Voluven structure is 0.4. From these properties, Voluven is usually presented as hydroxyethyl starch 130/0.4. Hetastarch is usually seen as 450/0.7; and pentastarch appears as 200/0.5.[11]

Voluven molecules are smaller than those of hetastarch and pentastarch, and the molecular decomposition of Voluven is faster. Thus, Voluven is likely excreted from the body faster and is less likely to cause plasma accumulation. These characteristics make Voluven less likely to cause the same undesirable effects as the other starches.[12]

A problem associated with HES is possible hemostasis impairment, specifically on vWF. However, the problem seems to be associated more with the higher substituted HES that have medium to high MW.[11] An increasing number of prospective studies have compared Voluven with other starches (**Table 2**).

Voluven was compared with the standard HES 200/0.5 (pentastarch) in 59 coronary artery bypass patients and was found to be similar in efficacy.[14] The mean infusion volume of HES was comparable between the 2 groups (2550 ± 561 mL in the group

Table 1
Single-dose pharmacokinetics of plasma expanders (data provided by Voluven Fresenius/ Hospira)

	Voluven (130/0.4)	Hespan (600/0.75)	Albumin
Clearance	17–31.4 mL/min	0.98 mL/min	—
Half-life	12–16 h	46.4 h	15 d
Elimination in urine	62% within 72 h	33% within 24 h 46% after 2 d 64% after 8 d	No renal elimination
Plasma concentrations of HES	14% of peak at 6 h <0.5 mg/mL in 24 h	10% of peak at 2 wk <0.5 mg/mL in 2 wk	—

Table 2
Investigations of Voluven (HES 130/0.4) compared with other colloids (HES 200/0.5, HES 670/0.75) or human albumin

Study: First Author, Year	Patient Population	Design	Number of Patients Enrolled	Outcomes
Gallandat Huet et al,[14] 2000	Cardiac surgery	Prospective, randomized, double-blinded, parallel-group, multicenter cohort	59	Compared HES 130/0.4 with HES 200/0.5 and found similar infusion volume requirements in both groups. A lower mean total blood loss was experienced with the HES 130/0.4 group and was reflected by a significantly lower use of packed RBCs
Jungheinrich et al,[12] 2002	Renal dysfunction	Prospective cohort	19	HES 130/0.4 total plasma clearance depended on renal function. Residual concentrations found 24 h after 500 mL were small, even in patients with severe renal dysfunction. C_{max} and terminal half-life were not dependent on renal function
Boldt et al,[15] 2007	Cardiac surgery with compromised renal function	Prospective, randomized cohort	50	Compared HES 130/0.4 with 5% human albumin to determine the effects of Voluven on renal function. No differences were seen in any of the outcome parameters after 48 h of volume resuscitation. The parameters examined included volumes infused on several markers of kidney function, serum creatinine, glomerular filtration rate, and cystatin C plasma levels. A 6-month follow-up showed that none of the patients developed acute renal failure
Gandhi et al,[11] 2007	Major orthopedic surgery	Prospective, controlled, randomized, double-blinded, multicenter cohort	100	Compared HES 130/0.4 with HES 670/0.75. No differences were found in fluid replacement volumes. Nadir factor VIII activity and vWF concentration was lower in hetastarch group than Voluven group within 2 h of end of surgery
Standl et al,[16] 2008	Pediatric, noncardiac surgery	Prospective, controlled, randomized, open, multicenter pilot cohort	82	Compared HES 130/0.4 with 5% human albumin. No differences in hemodynamics, coagulation profiles, fluid input or output, intensive care unit stay or length of hospital stay

receiving Voluven and 2446 ± 516 mL in the control group). Blood loss was found to be lower in patients receiving Voluven (1301 ± 551 mL) than in those receiving control (1821 ± 1222 mL), $P = 0.046$. This reduced blood loss was reflected in a lowered need for transfusion of packed red blood cells in patients receiving Voluven (241 ± 419 mL in the Voluven group versus 405 ± 757 mL in the control group). vWF increased to supranormal levels in both groups, but the increase was higher with Voluven.

In a study by Boldt and colleagues,[15] Voluven was compared with 5% human albumin to examine the effects on kidney function in a group of 50 patients who underwent coronary artery bypass. Voluven was given perioperatively until the second postoperative day to keep pulmonary artery occlusion pressure or central venous pressure between 12 and 14 mmHg. There were no significant differences with fluid input or output between the 2 groups. The use of diuretics and catecholamines, and hemodynamics were also comparable. Neither conventional measures of kidney function such as serum creatinine and glomerular filtration rate nor more sensitive measures such as cystatin C or kidney-specific proteins were significantly increased with Voluven compared with albumin. Sixty-day postoperative follow-ups showed no difference in kidney function between the Voluven and human albumin groups. There was also no difference in the occurrence of renal failure between the 2 groups.

The dependency on pharmacokinetics and the preservation of the volume effect of HES 130/0.4 on renal function were studied in 19 volunteers with nonanuric renal dysfunction.[12] These patients were given a single infusion of 500 mL of Voluven (HES 130/0.4) over 30 minutes. HES peak concentration and terminal half-life were not affected by renal impairment. The mean MW of HES in plasma showed lower values with increased renal impairment ($P = 0.04$). This study concluded that Voluven can be safely administered in patients with renal impairment, as long as urine flow is preserved, without plasma accumulation.[12]

The equivalence and efficacy of Voluven was compared with hetastarch (HES 670/0.75 in saline) in a study that investigated intravascular volume replacement therapy during major orthopedic surgery (with an expected blood loss of 500 mL or more) in 100 patients.[11] Colloid administration was guided by central venous pressure (CVP) and arterial blood pressure: infusion of colloids with CVP less than 10 mmHg, colloids administration or vasoactive agents used with CVP 10–15 mmHg and unacceptable blood pressure, and vasoactive agents administrated with CVP greater than 15 and unacceptable blood pressure. No colloids were infused after the end of surgery.

The primary end points included the total volume of colloid solution required during surgery (efficacy) and calculated total perioperative erythrocyte loss, nadir factor VIII activity and vWF antigen concentration within 2 hours of completion of surgery, and use of fresh frozen plasma (safety). Secondary end points were total fluid input and output and use of vasoactive drugs for efficacy, and hemodynamic stability and adverse events for safety.

In patients undergoing major orthopedic surgery (most involving the spine or hip), the mean volumes of colloids administered were similar in the 2 HES groups (1613 ± 778 mL in the Voluven group versus 1584 ± 958 mL in the control group).[11]

The nadir factor VIII activity within 2 hours of the end of surgery was lower for hetastarch than for Voluven ($P = .0499$), and a higher fraction of patients presented vWF values less than the lower limit 2 hours after surgery in the hetastarch group ($P = .027$). At 24 and 48 hours, values of factor VIII activity and vWF antigen were significantly higher for the Voluven group ($P<.0001$). Three serious coagulopathy events occurred in the hetastarch group, and none in the Voluven group.

In conclusion, this study showed that Voluven and hetastarch are equally effective plasma volume expanders, but Voluven has a lesser effect on coagulation.

In a prospective, controlled, randomized, open, multicenter pilot study, children younger than 2 years undergoing noncardiac surgery were treated with either Voluven (16.0 mL/kg) or human albumin 5% (16.9 mL/kg).[16] A total of 81 patients were treated and no differences in hemodynamics, coagulation parameters, or other laboratory values were detected between the 2 groups. Blood loss was significantly less in the group treated with albumin compared with the Voluven-treated group. However, there were no differences in the amount of red blood cells, fresh frozen plasma, or platelet concentrates between the groups. Albumin and Voluven were both effective for hemodynamic stabilization in pediatric noncardiac surgery, with no adverse impact on coagulation.[16]

In a recent study, 2 similar, low MW colloids were compared in 54 patients who underwent prolonged multilevel spinal surgeries (PLIF) involving 3 vertebrae or less. Voluven, previously regarded as the most benign toward coagulation, and a new saline-based HES, Hextend, were investigated.[17] Hextend (Biotime, United States) is a new type of HES with a physiologic pH and balanced electrolytes including calcium, which is beneficial to coagulation. For both groups, 15 mL/kg of solution were administered during surgery. Blood loss, coagulation, and electrolyte profiles were checked before infusion and 5 minutes, 3 hours, and 24 hours after infusion. The Hextend group showed slightly better electrolyte balance, however, more coagulation impairment and postoperative transfusions (37% vs 11%) compared with the Voluven group. The effect of Hextend on coagulation lasted until 24 hours after infusion. In conclusion, if coagulopathy is a concern during PLIF, then an HES with low MW/DS in a saline-based medium (Voluven) may be a better alternative than a HES with high MW/DS in a balanced salt medium (Hextend).

SUMMARY

Voluven is a new volume expander that can effectively replace fluids during major surgical procedures, has useful properties compared with albumin and the traditional hetastarch Hespan, and is more versatile for general clinical use.

REFERENCES

1. Morgan GE Jr, Mikhail MS, Murray MJ. Fluid management & transfusion. In: Foltin J, Lebowitz H, Boyle PJ, editors. Clinical anesthesiology. 4th edition. McGraw; 2006. p. 690–702.
2. Kaye AD, Riopelle JM. Intravascular fluid and electrolyte physiology. In: Miller RD, Eriksson LI, Fleisher LA, et al, editors. 7th edition, Miller's anesthesia, vol. 2. Philadelphia: Churchill Livingstone Elsevier; 2010. p. 1723–7.
3. Moss GS, Gould SA. Plasma expanders. An update. Am J Surg 1988;155(3): 425–34.
4. Pearson, Chris. Colloid and crystalloid resuscitation Intensive Care Unit. Wordpress.com, 23 January 2009. Available at: http://intensivecareunit.wordpress.com/2009/01/23/colloid-and-crystalloid-resuscitation/. Accessed 29 March, 2010.
5. Velanovich V. Crystalloid versus colloid fluid resuscitation: a meta-analysis of mortality. Surgery 1989;105(1):65–71.
6. Roth E, Lax LC, Maloney JV Jr. Ringer's lactate solution and extracellular fluid volume in the surgical patient: a critical analysis. Ann Surg 1969;169(2):149–64.

7. Mikura M, Yamaoka I, Doi M, et al. Glucose infusion suppresses surgery-induced muscle protein breakdown by inhibiting ubiquitin-proteasome pathway in rats. Anesthesiology 2009;110:81–8.

8. Alderson P, Bunn F, Lefebvre C, et al. Human albumin solution for resuscitation and volume expansion in critically ill patients. Cochrane Database Syst Rev 2004;4:CD00128.

9. Kozek-Langenecker SA. Effects of hydroxyethyl starch solutions on hemostasis. Anesthesiology 2005;103(3):654–60.

10. Mangar D, Gerson JI, Constantine RM, et al. Pulmonary edema and coagulopathy due to Hyskon (32% dextran-70) administration. Anesth Analg 1989;68(5):686–7.

11. Gandhi SD, Weiskopf RB, Jungheinrich C, et al. Volume replacement therapy during major orthopedic surgery using Voluven (hydroxyethyl starch 130/0.4) or hetastarch. Anesthesiology 2007;106(6):1120–7.

12. Jungheinrich C, Scharpf R, Wargenau M, et al. The pharmacokinetics and tolerability of an intravenous infusion of the new hydroxyethyl starch 130/0.4 (6%, 500 mL) in mild-to-severe renal impairment. Anesth Analg 2002;95(3): 544–51.

13. Approval memorandum – Voluven, December 20, 2007. US Food and Drug Administration. US Department of Health & Human Services, 2 February 2010. Available at: http://www.fda.gov/BiologicsBloodVaccines/BloodBloodProducts/ApprovedProducts/NewDrugApplicationsNDAs/ucm083364.htm. Accessed 29 March, 2010.

14. Gallandat Huet RC, Siemons AW, Baus D, et al. A novel hydroxyethyl starch (Voluven) for effective perioperative plasma volume substitution in cardiac surgery. Can J Anaesth 2000;47(12):1207–15.

15. Boldt J, Brosch C, Ducke M, et al. Influence of volume therapy with a modern hydroxyethylstarch preparation on kidney function in cardiac surgery patients with compromised renal function: a comparison with human albumin. Crit Care Med 2007;35(12):2740–6.

16. Standl T, Lochbuehler H, Galli C, et al. HES 130/0.4 (Voluven) or human albumin in children younger than 2 yr undergoing non-cardiac surgery. A prospective, randomized, open label, multicentre trial. Eur J Anaesthesiol 2008;25(6):437–45.

17. Choi SJ, Ahn HJ, Chung SS, et al. Hemostatic and electrolyte effects of hydroxyethyl starches in patients undergoing posterior lumbar interbody fusion using pedicle screws and cages. Spine (Phila Pa 1976) 2010;35(7):829–34.

Index

Note: Page numbers of article titles are in **boldface** type.

A

Advanced Cardiac Life Support (ACLS), amiodarone in, 540–541
Adverse effects, of amiodarone, 540
Alerts. *See* Real-time alerts.
Amiodarone, use by anesthesiologists in the OR and during CPR, **535–545**
    adverse effects of, 540
    as an antiarrhythmic, 539–540
    cardiac action potentials, 536
    history of, 539
    in ACLS, 540–541
    in cardiac surgery, 542–543
    sudden cardiac death, 535–536
    trials of, in sustained ventricular arrhythmias and cardiac arrest, 541–542
    Vaughan Williams classification, 537–538
    vs. lidocaine, procainaminde, and bretylium, 539
Anesthesia information management systems (AIMS), 355–483, 456–460
    anatomy of, **355–365**
        decision support, 361–362
            alerts and reminders, 362
            case templates, 362
        hardware component of, 357
        history of, 355–356
        integration with institutional electronic medical records, 363–364
        intraoperative record, 359–360
        key features and functionality of, 357–358
        overview, 355
        patient tracking, 363
        physiologic device interfaces, 358
        postoperative documentation, 360–361
        preoperative record, 359
        quality assurance, 361
        reporting for quality improvement, compliance, or research purposes, 362
        software component of, 356–357
        staff and billing information, 361
            automatic charge capture, 361
            staff concurrency checks, 361
    clinical research using, **377–388**
        clinician data entry, 386–387
        considerations in the US, 378–379
        creating a common structure, 381–384
        data quality considerations, 386

Anesthesiology Clin 29 (2011) 557–565
doi:10.1016/S1932-2275(11)00068-1
1932-2275/11/$ – see front matter © 2011 Elsevier Inc. All rights reserved.

Anesthesia (*continued*)
    informed consent, 379
    integrating complementary data sources, 379–381
    mapping structures to common concepts for multicenter research, 384–385
    multicenter perioperative outcomes group, 387–388
    novel record-linking technologies, 385–386
    overview, 377
    regulatory framework, 377–378
    researcher review of data, 387
    standardizing the format and mapping of data elements, 381
  creating a real return-on-investment for, **413–438**
    demonstrating meaningful use of EHR technology, 416–427
    hospital-based eligible professionals, 427
    implications for anesthesiologists, 427–433
    incentives for eligible professionals, 413–415
    opportunities for anesthesiologists, 433–438
  integration of the electronic health record (EHR) and, **455–483**
    benefits of an EHR, 461–465
    concerns about safety and usability of, 465–468
    effect on anesthesia workflows, 468–478
    EHR certification, 460–461
  marketplace and current vendors, **367–375**
    choices, 371–372
    listing of, 370
    non-AIMS vendors, 370
    process for making decision, 372–374
  quality improvement using, **439–454**
    benefits of electronic anesthesia data, 445–447
    benefits of that National Anesthesia Clinical Outcomes Registry (NACOR), 447–449
    data available, 441–442
    need for anesthesia outcomes data, 440–441
    potential pitfalls in the Anesthesia Quality Institute process, 449–451
    registry models, 442–445
  real-time alerts and reminders using, **389–396**
    clinical decision support, 390–392
    discussion and future directions, 394
    proof of concepts in peer-reviewed literature, 392–394
  shortcomings and challenges of adoption of, **397–412**
    cost barriers, 408–409
    cultural/organizational barriers, 409–410
    HIPPA Act and, 407
    technical barriers, 407–408
    with AIMS, 398–399
    with EMRs, 398
    with mobile computing, 399–407
      added value, 399–402
      informational tool or decision-making device, 405–406
      security, 406–407
      situational awareness, 402–405
      volume of data, 405
Anesthesia outcomes. *See* Outcomes, anesthesia.

Anesthesia Quality Institute, **439–454**
Anesthesia workflows. *See* Workflows, anesthesia.
Antiarrhythmics, amiodarone use by anesthesiologists in the OR and during CPR, **535–545**
    Vaughan Williams classification, 537–538

B

Billing information, in AIMS, 361
Bretylium, supplanted by amiodarone in ACLS and CPR protocols, 539

C

Cardiac action potentials, 536
Cardiac arrest, trials of amiodarone in, 541–542
Cardiac surgery, amiodarone in, 542–543
Cardiopulmonary bypass, alarm use after, using computerized clinical decision support systems, 393–394
Cardiopulmonary resuscitation (CPR), amiodarone use during, 535–545
Certification, of electronic health records, 460–461
Charge capture, automatic, in AIMS, 361
Clinical information systems, perioperative. *See* Anesthesia information management systems.
Clinical research. *See* Research, clinical.
Colloids, examples of, 550
    new (volvulen), 551–554
    versus crystalloids, 548
Communication, clinical, effect of electronic health records on, 470–472
    enhancing point-of-care vigilance using computers, 515
Compliance, reporting for, in AIMS, 362
Computerized practitioner order entry (CPOE), effect on anesthesia workflow, 473–474
Computers, in anesthesia, 485–531
    advanced integrated real-time displays, **487–504**
        action computation agent, 496–500
        challenges facing smart displays, 491–493
        challenges of alert-driven monitoring, 489–490
        effector method, 501
        electronic medical records for integrated patient monitoring, 490–491
        intelligent agents for advanced smart displays, 493–494
        patient monitoring and human in-the-loop controls, 488–489
        perception agent, 495–496
        Riskwatch integrated advanced smart display system, 494–495
    enhancing point of care vigilance using, **505–519**
        communication, 515
        impact on outcomes, 517
        information technology, 507–508
        safety and, 507–508
        situational awareness, 508–515
        smart systems and decision support, 515–517
    for perioperative simulation, **521–531**
        computer/web-based simulation training, 526–527
        immersive simulation technology, 522–525

Computers (*continued*)
     virtual reality, 525–526
Cost issues, as barrier to implementation of AIMS, 408–409
  creating a real return-on-investment for AIMS, **413–438**
    demonstrating meaningful use of EHR technology, 416–427
    hospital-based eligible professionals, 427
    implications for anesthesiologists, 427–433
    incentives for eligible professionals, 413–415
    opportunities for anesthesiologists, 433–438
Cost reduction, using computerized clinical decision support systems, 393
Critical care, use of computers for perioperative simulation in, **521–531**
Crystalloids, examples of, 548–549
  versus colloids, 548

D

Data entry, by clinicians to electronic medical records, value of for research purposes, 386–387
Death, sudden cardiac, 535–536
Decision support, advanced integrated real-time clinical displays, **482–504**
  enhancing point-of-care vigilance using smart systems, 515–517
  in anesthesia information management systems, 361–362
    alerts and reminders, 362, **389–396**
    effect on anesthesia workflow, 474–475
Devices, medical, interface with, in AIMS, 358
Displays, clinical, advanced integrated real-time, **482–504**
Documentation, in electronic health records, effect on anesthesia workflow, 470–472
    intraoperative, 359–360
    postoperative, 360–361
    preoperative, 359
Drug dosing reminders, using computerized clinical decision support systems, 392
Drug-drug interactions, using computerized clinical decision support systems, 393

E

Electronic health records (EHRs). *See* Electronic medical records (EMRs).
Electronic medical records (EMRs), clinical research using, **377–388**
    clinician data entry, 386–387
    considerations in the US, 378–379
    creating a common structure, 381–384
    data quality considerations, 386
    informed consent, 379
    integrating complementary data sources, 379–381
    mapping structures to common concepts for multicenter research, 384–385
    multicenter perioperative outcomes group, 387–388
    novel record-linking technologies, 385–386
    overview, 377
    regulatory framework, 377–378
    researcher review of data, 387
    standardizing the format and mapping of data elements, 381
  for integrated patient monitoring, 490–491

integration of AIMS and, **455–483**
    benefits of, 461–465
    certification, 460–461
    concerns about safety and usability of, 465–468
    effect on anesthesia workflows, 468–478
        clinical communication and documentation, 470–472
        clinical decision support, 474–475
        computerized practitioner order entry (CPOE), 473–474
        infrastructure, support, and downtime, 476–477
        integration and interoperability, 472
        patient admission, discharge, transfer, location, and outpatient status, 475–476
        security/authorization, 472–473
        sharing and integration, 469–470
        support, troubleshooting, fixes, and upgrades, 477–478
    shortcomings with, 398

F

Fluid replacement, with volvulen, **547–555**

H

Hardware, in AIMS, 357
Health Information Technology or Economic and Clinical Health (HITECH) Act, 456–460
    creating a real return-on-investment for information systems after, **413–438**
        demonstrating meaningful use of EHR technology, 416–427
        hospital-based eligible professionals, 427
        implications for anesthesiologists, 427–433
        incentives for eligible professionals, 413–415
        opportunities for anesthesiologists, 433–438
Health Insurance Portability and Accountability Act, mobile computing and, 407
Hydroxyethyl starch (HES), new colloid solution volvulen, **547–555**

I

Immersive simulation technology, for perioperative simulation, 522–525
Implementation, of AIMS, shortcomings and challenges of, **397-412**
Information technology, 355–555
    anesthesia information management systems (AIMS), 355–483
        anatomy of, **355–365**
        clinical research using, **377–388**
        creating a real return-on-investment for, **413–438**
        integration of the electronic health record and, **455–483**
        marketplace and current vendors, **367–375**
        quality improvement using, **439–454**
        real-time alerts and reminders using, **389–396**
        shortcomings and challenges of adoption of, **397–412**
    computers in anesthesia, 485–531
        advanced integrated real-time displays, **487–504**
        enhancing point of care vigilance using, **505–519**
        for perioperative simulation, **521–531**

Informed consent, to use data from electronic medical records for research purposes, 379
Intraoperative documentation, in AIMS, 359–360

L

Lidocaine, supplanted by amiodarone in ACLS and CPR protocols, 539
Location, patient, within the hospital, tracking with AIMS, 475–476

M

Market penetration, for AIMS, **367–375**
Medical devices, interface with, in AIMS, 358
Mobile computing. *See also* Anesthesia information management systems (AIMS).
    challenges of, 399–407
        added value, 399–402
        informational tool or decision-making device, 405–406
        security, 406–407
        situational awareness, 402–405
        volume of data, 405
Monitoring, patient, advanced integrated real-time displays, **487–504**
        action computation agent, 496–500
        challenges facing smart displays, 491–493
        challenges of alert-driven monitoring, 489–490
        effector method, 501
        electronic medical records for integrated patient monitoring, 490–491
        intelligent agents for advanced smart displays, 493–494
        patient monitoring and human in-the-loop controls, 488–489
        perception agent, 495–496
        Riskwatch integrated advanced smart display system, 494–495
Multicenter Perioperative Outcomes Group, 387–388

N

National Anesthesia Clinical Outcomes Registry (NACOR), quality improvement using,
    439–454

O

Observational research. *See* Research, clinical.
Organizational barriers, to implementation of AIMS, 409-410
Outcomes, anesthesia, impact of enhanced point-of-care vigilance using computers, 517
    quality improvement using automated data sources, **439–454**
        benefits of electronic anesthesia data, 445–447
        benefits of the National Anesthesia Clinical Outcomes Registry (NACOR), 447–449
        data available, 441–442
        need for anesthesia outcomes data, 440–441
        potential pitfalls in the Anesthesia Quality Institute process, 449–451
        registry models, 442–445

P

Pain medicine, use of computers for perioperative simulation in, **521–531**
Patient monitoring. *See* Monitoring *and* Vigilance.
Perioperative clinical information systems. *See* Anesthesia information management systems.
Perioperative medicine, clinical research on, using electronic medical records, **377–388**
Physiologic devices, interface with, in AIMS, 358
Postoperative documentation, in AIMS, 360–361
Postoperative nausea and vomiting, reminders for adherence to guidelines for using computerized clinical decision support systems, 393
Preoperative documentation, in AIMS, 359
Procainamide, supplanted by amiodarone in ACLS and CPR protocols, 539

Q

Quality assurance, in AIMS, 361
Quality improvement, reporting for, in AIMS, 362
    using automated data sources, **439–454**
        benefits of electronic anesthesia data, 445–447
        benefits of the National Anesthesia Clinical Outcomes Registry (NACOR), 447–449
        data available, 441–442
        need for anesthesia outcomes data, 440–441
        potential pitfalls in the Anesthesia Quality Institute process, 449–451
        registry models, 442–445
    with integration of the electronic health record and AIMS, **455–483**

R

Real-time alerts, challenges of alert-driven monitoring, 489–490
    in health care, using information systems for, **389–396**
Registries, anesthesia, benefits of the National Anesthesia Clinical Outcomes Registry (NACOR), 447–449
    models for, 442–445
Reminders, in health care, using information systems for, **389–396**
Research, clinical, using electronic medical records, **377–388**
        clinician data entry, 386–387
        considerations in the US, 378–379
        creating a common structure, 381–384
        data quality considerations, 386
        informed consent, 379
        integrating complementary data sources, 379–381
        mapping structures to common concepts for multicenter research, 384–385
        multicenter perioperative outcomes group, 387–388
        novel record-linking technologies, 385–386
        overview, 377
        regulatory framework, 377–378
        researcher review of data, 387
        standardizing the format and mapping of data elements, 381
    reporting for, in AIMS, 362
Return-on-investment. *See* Cost issues.

Revenue capture, using computerized clinical decision support systems, 393
Riskwatch integrated advanced smart display system, 494–495

S

Safety, patient, advanced integrated real-time clinical displays, **482–504**
    enhancing point-of-care vigilance using computers, **505–519**
        communication, 515
        impact on outcomes, 517
        information technology, 507–508
        safety and, 507–508
        situational awareness, 508–515
        smart systems and decision support, 515–517
Security, issues with mobile computing, 406–407
    of electronic health records, 465–468, 472–473
Simulation, perioperative, use of computers in anesthesia, critical care, and pain medicine, **521–531**
        computer/web-based simulation training, 526–527
        immersive simulation technology, 522–525
        virtual reality, 525–526
Situational awareness, enhancing point-of-care vigilance using computers, 508–512
        in the operating room, 512–513
        in the operating suite, 513–514
    with mobile computing, 402–405
Smart systems, and decision support, enhancing point-of-care vigilance using, 515–517
        challenges facing smart displays, 491–493
        intelligent agents for advanced displays, 493–494
        Riskwatch integrated advanced smart display system, 494–495
Software, in AIMS, 356–357
Staff concurrency checks, in AIMS, 361
Sudden cardiac death, 535–536

T

Tachyarrhythmias, trials of amiodarone in sustained ventricular, 541–542
Tracking, patient, reporting for, in AIMS, 363
Training, medical, use of computers for perioperative simulation, **521–531**

V

Vaughan Williams classification, of antiarrhythmic drugs, 537–538
Vendors, for AIMS, **367–375**
        choices, 371–372
        listing of, 370
        non-AIMS vendors, 370
        process for making decision, 372–374
Ventricular tachyarrhythmias, trials of amiodarone in sustained, 541–542
Vigilance, point-of-care, enhancement of using computers, **505–519**
        communication, 515
        impact on outcomes, 517
        information technology, 507–508

safety and, 507–508
    situational awareness, 508–515
    smart systems and decision support, 515–517
Virtual reality, perioperative simulation using, 525–526
Volvulen, new colloid solution, **547–555**
    colloid *vs.* crystalloids, 548
    colloids, examples of, 549–554
    crystalloids, examples of, 548–549
    fluid replacement, 548

W

Web-based simulation training, 526–527
Workflows, anesthesia, effect of electronic health records on, 468–478
    clinical communication and documentation, 470–472
    clinical decision support, 474–475
    computerized practitioner order entry (CPOE), 473–474
    infrastructure, support, and downtime, 476–477
    integration and interoperability, 472
    patient admission, discharge, transfer, location, and outpatient status, 475–476
    security/authorization, 472–473
    sharing and integration, 469–470
    support, troubleshooting, fixes, and upgrades, 477–478

Moving?

Make sure your subscription moves with you!

To notify us of your new address, find your **Clinics Account Number** (located on your mailing label above your name), and contact customer service at:

Email: journalscustomerservice-usa@elsevier.com

800-654-2452 (subscribers in the U.S. & Canada)
314-447-8871 (subscribers outside of the U.S. & Canada)

Fax number: 314-447-8029

Elsevier Health Sciences Division
Subscription Customer Service
3251 Riverport Lane
Maryland Heights, MO 63043

*To ensure uninterrupted delivery of your subscription, please notify us at least 4 weeks in advance of move.

Printed and bound by CPI Group (UK) Ltd, Croydon, CR0 4YY

03/10/2024

01040454-0003